The Herbal Natural Plant Power Tablets Book:

Your Complete Guide to Natural Healing

Table of Contents

Introduction

The Power of Herbal Tablets

Herbal tablets are a remarkable fusion of ancient wisdom and modern convenience, offering a potent and practical way to harness the healing properties of plants. Their power lies in their ability to concentrate the benefits of medicinal herbs into a compact, easy-to-use form, providing a host of advantages for those seeking natural health solutions.

1. Concentrated Healing: Herbal tablets are designed to encapsulate the therapeutic properties of herbs in a concentrated format. By carefully extracting and processing the active components of plants, tablets deliver a potent dose of natural medicine with each serving. This concentration ensures that you receive the maximum benefits from the herbs, making tablets a powerful option for addressing various health concerns.

2. Precision and Consistency: One of the key advantages of herbal tablets is their precision in dosage. Unlike teas or tinctures, tablets offer a standardized amount of herbal extract in each dose, allowing for consistent and reliable effects. This precision helps in managing specific health issues effectively and ensures that you know exactly how much of the herb you are consuming.

3. Portability and Convenience: Herbal tablets are incredibly convenient for on-the-go use. They are easy to carry, store, and take whenever needed, making them an ideal choice for busy lifestyles. Whether you're at work, traveling, or simply need a quick remedy, tablets provide a portable and practical solution for maintaining your health.

4. Long Shelf Life: Compared to fresh herbs or liquid extracts, herbal tablets have a longer shelf life. Their solid form helps preserve the potency of the herbal ingredients, allowing you to keep a stock of remedies without worrying about spoilage. Properly stored tablets can remain effective for extended periods, ensuring that you always have access to your preferred remedies.

5. Customizable and Versatile: Creating your own herbal tablets offers the flexibility to tailor remedies to your specific needs. You can combine different herbs to address multiple health issues, adjust dosages to suit your personal requirements, and experiment with various formulations. This versatility allows you to create personalized remedies that align with your health goals and preferences.

6. Holistic Benefits: Herbal tablets are not just about alleviating symptoms; they aim to support overall wellness by addressing the root causes of health issues. Many herbal remedies work synergistically to enhance your body's natural healing processes, promote balance, and strengthen your immune system. By focusing on holistic health, herbal tablets help you achieve long-term well-being rather than just temporary relief.

In summary, the power of herbal tablets lies in their ability to deliver concentrated, precise, and convenient natural remedies. Whether you're new to herbal medicine or a seasoned practitioner, incorporating herbal tablets into your health regimen can provide a valuable and effective means of supporting your overall wellness and addressing a range of health concerns.

Benefits of Using Herbal Tablets for Natural Healing

Herbal tablets are more than just a modern convenience; they offer a range of benefits that make them an appealing choice for natural healing. Their unique attributes combine the efficacy of traditional herbal medicine with the practicality of contemporary delivery methods. Here's how herbal tablets can enhance your journey towards better health:

1. **Effective and Concentrated Formulas: Herbal tablets concentrate the active ingredients of medicinal herbs into a small, potent dose. This allows you to receive the full therapeutic benefits of the herbs in a controlled and consistent manner, ensuring that you get the maximum efficacy from each dose.

2. **Ease of Use: Tablets are incredibly user-friendly. They eliminate the need for preparation and measuring, making it easy to integrate them into your daily routine. With just a simple swallow, you can benefit from the healing properties of herbs without the hassle of brewing teas or mixing tinctures.

3. **Consistent Dosage: Unlike other forms of herbal remedies, such as teas or powders, tablets provide a precise and consistent dosage of herbal extracts. This precision helps in managing specific health concerns more effectively and ensures that you are getting a reliable amount of the herbal components with each dose.

4. **Portability and Convenience: Herbal tablets are easy to carry and store, making them ideal for busy lifestyles. Whether you're traveling, working, or simply need a quick remedy, tablets offer a convenient solution that can be taken anytime, anywhere. Their compact nature ensures that you have access to natural healing no matter where life takes you.

5. **Long Shelf Life: Herbal tablets generally have a longer shelf life compared to fresh herbs or liquid extracts. Their solid form helps in preserving the potency of the herbal ingredients, reducing the risk of spoilage and ensuring that your remedies remain effective for extended periods.

6. **Customizable Formulations: Creating your own herbal tablets allows you to tailor remedies to your specific needs. You can combine various herbs to address multiple health concerns, adjust dosages according to your personal requirements, and experiment with different formulations to find what works best for you.

7. **Holistic Health Support: Herbal tablets often address the root causes of health issues rather than just alleviating symptoms. Many herbal remedies work synergistically to support overall wellness, strengthen the immune system, and promote balance in the body. This holistic approach helps in achieving long-term health benefits and maintaining well-being.

8. **Minimal Side Effects: When used correctly, herbal tablets generally have fewer side effects compared to synthetic medications. Many herbs have a long history of safe use and are well-tolerated by most people. This makes herbal tablets a gentle alternative for those looking to avoid the adverse effects often associated with conventional drugs.

9. **Affordability: Herbal tablets can be a cost-effective option for natural healing. By making your own tablets, you can save money on expensive store-bought remedies and ensure that you are using high-quality, fresh ingredients. Additionally, many herbs are readily available and affordable, making it easier to maintain a natural health regimen without breaking the bank.

In conclusion, herbal tablets offer a range of benefits that make them a valuable addition to any natural healing practice. Their effectiveness, ease of use, and versatility combine to provide a practical and potent means of supporting your health and well-being. By incorporating herbal tablets into your daily routine, you can experience the full potential of herbal medicine and enjoy a more balanced and healthful life.

How to Use This Book

Welcome to your journey into the world of herbal tablets! This book is designed to be a comprehensive guide to creating and using herbal tablets for natural healing. Here's how to navigate and make the most of the information and resources provided:

1. **Start with the Basics: Begin by familiarizing yourself with the foundational concepts of herbal medicine and tablet-making. **Chapter 1** provides an overview of herbal medicine's history and principles, while

Chapter 2 covers the essential tools, ingredients, and techniques you'll need to get started.

2. Understand Tablet Formulations: In **Chapter 3, you'll learn about the principles of herbal tablet formulations, including how to determine dosages, select binding agents, and ensure the stability and potency of your tablets. This knowledge is crucial for creating effective and safe remedies.

**3. Explore Remedy Recipes: Chapter 4 is dedicated to a wide range of remedy recipes for common health issues. Each section focuses on specific health concerns, such as immune support, digestive health, stress relief, and pain management. Use these recipes as a starting point to create tablets tailored to your needs.

**4. Dive into Specialized Tablets: Chapter 5 covers specialized herbal tablets for various health conditions, including respiratory health, cardiovascular support, skin care, hormonal balance, and cognitive function. This chapter offers additional recipes and formulations for more targeted health support.

5. Master Advanced Techniques: Once you're comfortable with the basics, **Chapter 6 introduces advanced techniques and tips for customizing your herbal tablets. Learn how to blend herbs for enhanced effects, troubleshoot common issues, and refine your tablet-making process.

6. Incorporate Tablets into Daily Life: Chapter 7 provides guidance on integrating herbal tablets into your daily health regimen. Discover how to create a personal tablet routine, combine tablets with other natural remedies, and read inspiring case studies of successful herbal tablet use.

7. Utilize Resources and Further Reading: Chapter 8 offers additional resources for expanding your herbal knowledge. Find recommended books, online resources, and directories for sourcing quality herbs and supplies.

8. Refer to Appendices: The appendices include a glossary of herbal terms, an herb identification guide, and an index of herbal tablet recipes. These resources are valuable for quick reference and deeper understanding of the material covered in the book.

9. Experiment and Personalize: Feel free to experiment with the recipes and techniques provided. Herbal medicine is a versatile and evolving field, and personalizing your approach can yield the best results. Trust your intuition and adjust formulations to fit your unique health needs.

By following these guidelines, you'll be well-equipped to explore the world of herbal tablets and harness their natural healing powers. Whether you're a beginner or an experienced herbalist, this book aims to provide you with practical knowledge and tools to support your health and well-being through the art of tablet-making.

Chapter 1: Understanding Herbal Medicine

The Basics of Herbal Medicine

Herbal medicine is a time-honored practice that utilizes plants and plant-derived substances to enhance health, prevent illness, and address various conditions. This section explores the fundamental elements of herbal medicine, providing a foundation for creating and using herbal tablets effectively.

Herbs and Plant Parts

Herbs used in medicinal applications come from various parts of plants, each offering distinct properties and benefits.

- **Leaves** are often valued for their essential oils and antioxidants. Herbs like peppermint and basil are known for their refreshing and supportive effects on health.

- **Flowers** are typically used for their soothing and calming qualities. Chamomile and calendula are examples of flowers that help with relaxation and skin health.

- **Roots** are rich in potent compounds and are often used for their strong therapeutic effects. Ginger and ginseng are well-known for their anti-inflammatory and immune-boosting properties.

- **Bark** contains concentrated compounds that can support various health functions. Examples include cinnamon bark for its digestive benefits and slippery elm for soothing the digestive tract.

- **Seeds** are often used for their nutrient content and specific health benefits. Flaxseeds and fenugreek are examples that support cardiovascular and digestive health.

- **Fruits** provide vitamins and antioxidants beneficial for health. Elderberries and rose hips are known for their immune-boosting and antioxidant-rich properties.

Active Compounds

Plants contain a diverse range of active compounds that contribute to their medicinal effects:

- **Alkaloids** are known for their strong physiological effects and can offer relief from pain and inflammation. Morphine from the opium poppy and caffeine from coffee beans are notable examples.

- **Flavonoids** provide antioxidant and anti-inflammatory benefits, helping to combat oxidative stress. Examples include quercetin from onions and catechins from green tea.

- **Glycosides** are compounds that can offer therapeutic benefits, particularly in cardiovascular health. Digitoxin from foxglove and saponins from ginseng are key examples.

- **Essential Oils** are aromatic compounds that provide therapeutic benefits such as relaxation and antimicrobial effects. Lavender oil and eucalyptus oil are commonly used for their calming and decongestant properties.

Preparation Methods

Herbal remedies can be prepared in various forms, each with its own advantages:

- **Teas** are made by steeping herbs in hot water, extracting water-soluble compounds. They offer a gentle remedy and are commonly used with herbs like chamomile and peppermint.

- **Tinctures** are concentrated extracts made by soaking herbs in alcohol or vinegar. They are effective for preserving and intensifying active compounds, with examples like echinacea and valerian root tinctures.

- **Extracts** are concentrated solutions that use solvents to extract active ingredients. Standardized extracts such as ginkgo biloba and St. John's wort provide consistent potency for specific health benefits.

- **Capsules and Tablets** contain powdered or concentrated herbal extracts, offering a convenient and precise way to take herbal remedies. Turmeric capsules and milk thistle tablets are examples of their use for anti-inflammatory and liver-supporting purposes.

Dosage and Potency

Accurate dosage is essential for the effectiveness and safety of herbal remedies:

- Different forms of herbal preparations have varying concentrations and potencies. Teas generally have lower concentrations compared to tinctures and extracts.

- Standardization of herbal products ensures consistent potency, especially for extracts and capsules. This helps in achieving reliable therapeutic effects.

- Dosage should be adjusted based on individual needs and responses. Starting with lower doses and gradually increasing, if needed, allows for safe and effective use.

Safety and Quality

Ensuring the safety and quality of herbal medicine is crucial:

- **Source and Purity**: Use herbs from reputable sources to avoid contaminants and ensure efficacy. Organic and wildcrafted herbs are often preferred.

- **Interactions**: Be mindful of potential interactions between herbs and medications. Consult with a healthcare provider if taking prescription drugs or if you have underlying health conditions.

- **Allergies and Sensitivities**: Test for allergies or sensitivities to specific herbs before regular use. Discontinue use if any adverse reactions occur.

Understanding these basics of herbal medicine—including the types of plant parts used, active compounds, preparation methods, dosage considerations, and safety practices—will provide a solid foundation for creating effective and safe herbal tablets. This knowledge will empower you to harness the full potential of herbal remedies and integrate them effectively into your health regimen.

History and Traditional Uses

Herbal medicine has been an integral part of human health and healing practices for millennia. Its rich history spans various cultures and civilizations, each contributing unique perspectives and practices to the art of using plants for health. Understanding the historical and traditional uses of herbal medicine provides valuable insights into its continued relevance and efficacy today.

Ancient Traditions

The use of herbs for medicinal purposes dates back to ancient civilizations, where plants were a primary source of healing. In ancient Egypt, herbal medicine was well-developed, with records such as the Ebers Papyrus documenting over 700 remedies, including herbs like garlic and juniper. The Egyptians used herbs for both internal and external ailments, combining them with rituals and spiritual practices.

In ancient China, herbal medicine evolved into a sophisticated system known as Traditional Chinese Medicine (TCM). TCM emphasizes balance and harmony within the body, guided by the principles of Qi (vital energy) and the interplay of Yin and Yang. Herbal formulas in TCM were crafted to restore balance and address imbalances within the body's systems. Key texts like the "Shennong Ben Cao Jing" (Divine Farmer's Materia Medica) detail a comprehensive array of herbs and their uses.

In India, Ayurveda developed as a holistic approach to health that focuses on balancing the three doshas—Vata, Pitta, and Kapha. Ayurveda incorporates herbs into its treatments, emphasizing the importance of personalized remedies based on individual constitution and imbalances. Ancient texts like the "Charaka Samhita" and "Sushruta Samhita" provide extensive knowledge about herbal medicines and their applications.

Traditional Chinese Medicine (TCM)

Traditional Chinese Medicine (TCM) has a long and rich history, with its roots tracing back over 2,000 years. TCM operates on the concept that health is a balance of Qi (vital energy), and imbalances can lead to illness. Herbs are used in TCM to restore this balance and treat various health conditions.

Formulas in TCM are often complex, combining multiple herbs to create a synergistic effect. Each herb in a formula is chosen based on its properties, such as warming or cooling effects, and its ability to interact harmoniously with other herbs. Common TCM herbs include ginseng for energy, ginger for digestion, and licorice root for harmonizing other herbs in a formula.

Ayurveda

Ayurveda, the traditional system of medicine from India, focuses on maintaining health by balancing the body's three doshas: Vata, Pitta, and Kapha. Each dosha represents different aspects of physiological and psychological functions, and imbalance in these doshas can lead to illness.

Herbs in Ayurveda are used to restore balance to the doshas and support overall health. Remedies are tailored to an individual's specific dosha and current state of health. For example, ashwagandha is used to support vitality and reduce stress, while turmeric is valued for its anti-inflammatory properties. Ayurvedic texts like the "Charaka Samhita" and "Sushruta Samhita" offer extensive knowledge about herbal remedies and their uses in maintaining health and treating disease.

Western Herbalism

Western herbalism has its origins in the traditional practices of indigenous cultures and early European herbalists. This approach often emphasizes the use of local plants and the natural healing abilities of the body.

In Europe, herbal medicine was practiced by herbalists and folk healers who used plants to treat a wide range of ailments. This knowledge was passed down through generations and compiled in texts such as Nicholas Culpeper's "The English Physician," which detailed the medicinal uses of common herbs.

In North America, indigenous peoples utilized a vast array of native plants for medicinal purposes. Their knowledge was closely tied to their environment and spiritual practices. The use of herbs like echinacea and goldenseal by Native American tribes is an example of this deep connection to plants and their healing properties.

Modern Applications

Herbal medicine continues to be relevant in the modern era, blending traditional wisdom with contemporary research. Many herbal practices from ancient traditions have been validated by scientific studies, leading to their integration into complementary and integrative medicine.

In today's health landscape, herbal remedies are often used alongside conventional treatments to enhance overall well-being and support specific health conditions. This integrative approach allows individuals to benefit from both traditional herbal knowledge and modern medical advancements.

Understanding the history and traditional uses of herbal medicine offers valuable insights into its continued relevance and application. By learning from these rich traditions, we can better appreciate the depth and breadth of herbal remedies and their role in promoting health and healing.

Modern Applications and Benefits

In contemporary times, herbal medicine has evolved from its traditional roots to become an integral part of modern healthcare. Its applications are diverse, ranging from preventive health measures to complementary treatments for various conditions. Understanding the modern applications and benefits of herbal medicine highlights its relevance and effectiveness in today's health landscape.

Integrative and Complementary Medicine

Herbal medicine is increasingly used alongside conventional medical treatments in integrative and complementary medicine. This approach combines the strengths of both traditional and modern practices to provide a holistic care strategy.

- **Supporting Conventional Treatments**: Herbal remedies are often used to support and enhance the effectiveness of conventional treatments. For instance, ginger and turmeric are commonly used to alleviate nausea and inflammation associated with chemotherapy, while valerian root can aid in managing anxiety and sleep disturbances often experienced by patients undergoing medical treatments.

- **Managing Chronic Conditions**: Herbal medicine plays a significant role in managing chronic conditions such as arthritis, diabetes, and cardiovascular diseases. Herbs like turmeric and boswellia are known for their anti-inflammatory properties, which can help reduce joint pain and inflammation in arthritis. Cinnamon and fenugreek are used to support healthy blood sugar levels in diabetes management.

- **Enhancing Overall Wellness**: Many individuals use herbal supplements to promote general well-being and prevent illness. Adaptogenic herbs like ashwagandha and rhodiola are valued for their ability to enhance resilience to stress and support overall vitality.

Evidence-Based Research

Modern science has begun to validate the effectiveness of many herbal remedies through rigorous research. This evidence-based approach helps bridge the gap between traditional herbal practices and contemporary medical standards.

- **Clinical Studies**: Numerous clinical studies have investigated the efficacy of herbal remedies for various health conditions. For example, studies have demonstrated that St. John's wort can be effective in managing mild to moderate depression, while echinacea may reduce the duration and severity of cold symptoms.

- **Standardization and Quality Control**: Advances in herbal medicine include efforts to standardize herbal extracts and ensure consistent quality. Standardization involves ensuring that herbal products contain specific concentrations of active ingredients, which enhances their reliability and effectiveness. This approach helps in producing consistent and potent herbal supplements.

- **Safety Assessments**: Modern research also focuses on assessing the safety of herbal remedies, including potential interactions with medications and side effects. This research contributes to safer use of herbs and helps consumers make informed decisions.

Personalized Medicine

The concept of personalized medicine, which tailors treatments to individual genetic and health profiles, is increasingly being applied to herbal medicine.

- **Tailoring Remedies**: Personalized herbal medicine involves selecting and customizing herbal remedies based on individual health conditions, genetic factors, and lifestyle. For example, herbal formulations can be adjusted to address specific symptoms or health concerns unique to the individual, enhancing their effectiveness.

- **Integrating Lifestyle Factors**: Personalized herbal medicine also considers lifestyle factors such as diet, exercise, and stress levels. Herbs can be chosen to complement an individual's lifestyle and address specific needs, such as using adaptogens to support stress management or incorporating herbs that promote digestive health.

Sustainable and Ethical Practices

Modern applications of herbal medicine also emphasize sustainability and ethical practices, ensuring that the use of herbs is environmentally responsible and socially equitable.

- **Sustainable Harvesting**: Efforts are being made to ensure that herbal plants are harvested sustainably, preserving natural ecosystems and preventing overexploitation. Sustainable harvesting practices help maintain the availability of medicinal plants for future generations.

- **Ethical Sourcing**: Ethical sourcing involves ensuring that herbal products are obtained from reputable suppliers who follow fair trade practices. This includes supporting local communities and ensuring fair compensation for those involved in the cultivation and harvesting of medicinal plants.

Education and Empowerment

Herbal medicine empowers individuals to take an active role in their health by providing them with knowledge and tools to use herbal remedies effectively.

- **Educational Resources**: Modern education on herbal medicine includes resources such as books, online courses, and workshops. These resources help individuals learn about the benefits, uses, and safety of herbal remedies, enabling them to make informed choices about their health.

- **Self-Care Practices**: Incorporating herbal medicine into self-care routines can enhance overall well-being. Simple practices such as making herbal teas, creating tinctures, and using essential oils can support daily health and promote a holistic approach to self-care.

In summary, modern applications of herbal medicine reflect a blend of traditional wisdom and contemporary research. Its benefits include supporting conventional treatments, managing chronic conditions, enhancing overall wellness, and embracing personalized and sustainable practices. By integrating evidence-based research and ethical considerations, herbal medicine continues to be a valuable and relevant component of modern healthcare.

Chapter 2: Getting Started with Herbal Tablets

Essential Tools and Equipment

Creating herbal tablets requires a range of tools and equipment to ensure precision, consistency, and quality. This section outlines the essential tools and equipment needed for the process, from preparing herbal extracts to forming and storing the tablets.

Herbal Preparation Tools

Before forming tablets, herbs need to be processed into usable forms, such as powders or extracts. The following tools are essential for these initial steps:

- **Herb Grinder or Mill**: A high-quality herb grinder or mill is crucial for turning dried herbs into fine powders. This ensures that the active compounds are evenly distributed in the tablets. Choose a grinder that can handle various herb types and achieve a consistent particle size.

- **Sieve or Screen**: A sieve or screen is used to further refine the powdered herbs, removing any larger particles that could affect tablet consistency. Fine mesh sieves are typically used to ensure a smooth powder.

- **Mortar and Pestle**: For small-scale preparations, a mortar and pestle can be used to crush and grind herbs manually. This tool is particularly useful for fresh herbs or when preparing small batches.

Extraction Equipment

To concentrate the active ingredients from herbs, extraction methods are employed. The following equipment is used for different types of herbal extractions:

- **Tincture Makers**: For alcohol-based extractions, tincture makers or jars with tight-sealing lids are used. These containers allow herbs to steep in alcohol or vinegar, extracting their active compounds over time.

- **Decoction Pots**: For boiling herbs to create decoctions, a sturdy pot or saucepan is needed. It should be made of non-reactive material, such as stainless steel, to avoid any chemical reactions with the herbs.

- **Infusion Pitchers**: For preparing herbal infusions, a heat-resistant pitcher or teapot can be used. Infusion pitchers are typically made of glass or ceramic and are suitable for steeping herbs in hot water.

- **Filtration Tools**: After extraction, herbs need to be filtered to remove solid particles. Cheesecloth, coffee filters, or fine mesh strainers are commonly used to strain tinctures and infusions.

Tablet Formulation Tools

Formulating and pressing herbal tablets requires specific tools to ensure uniformity and quality:

- **Tablet Press**: A tablet press is an essential tool for creating consistent and uniform tablets. It compresses the powdered herb mixture and excipients into tablet form. There are manual and automatic presses available, depending on the scale of production.

- **Tablet Molds**: For small-scale or homemade tablet production, tablet molds can be used. These molds come in various sizes and shapes, allowing you to create tablets according to your preferences.

- **Mixing Bowls and Spatulas**: Mixing bowls and spatulas are used to combine the herbal powders and excipients thoroughly before pressing them into tablets. Ensure that the mixing bowls are clean and suitable for handling herbal materials.

- **Weighing Scales**: Accurate dosing requires precise measurement of herbs and excipients. A high-quality digital weighing scale is essential for measuring ingredients accurately and ensuring the correct dosage in each tablet.

Quality Control Tools

Maintaining the quality and safety of herbal tablets involves monitoring various factors:

- **Microscope**: A microscope can be used to examine the texture and consistency of the powdered herbs and finished tablets. This helps ensure that the herbs are properly ground and that tablets are uniform in size.

- **Tablet Hardness Tester**: This tool measures the hardness and disintegration of tablets to ensure they meet quality standards. Proper hardness is crucial for the tablet's dissolution and effectiveness.

- **pH Meter**: For certain herbal formulations, especially those involving acidic or alkaline extracts, a pH meter can be used to measure and adjust the pH levels to ensure optimal stability and effectiveness.

Storage Solutions

Proper storage is essential for maintaining the potency and longevity of herbal tablets:

- **Airtight Containers**: Store tablets in airtight containers to protect them from moisture, light, and air. Glass jars with tight-sealing lids or high-quality plastic containers are suitable options.

- **Cool, Dry Storage**: Keep containers in a cool, dry place to prevent degradation of the active compounds. Avoid storing tablets in areas with high humidity or direct sunlight.

- **Labeling Supplies**: Clearly label all containers with information about the contents, dosage, and expiration date. Use waterproof and durable labels to ensure that information remains legible over time.

Safety and Hygiene

Maintaining safety and hygiene is crucial throughout the process:

- **Cleaning Supplies**: Keep all tools and equipment clean and free from contaminants. Use non-toxic cleaning agents and ensure thorough rinsing and drying of equipment.

- **Personal Protective Equipment (PPE)**: Wear gloves, masks, and protective eyewear when handling herbs and extracts to prevent contamination and exposure to potential allergens or irritants.

By equipping yourself with the essential tools and equipment outlined in this section, you can effectively create and manage high-quality herbal tablets. Proper preparation, formulation, and storage practices contribute to the overall success and safety of your herbal medicine endeavors.

Ingredients: Choosing Quality Herbs

Selecting high-quality herbs is fundamental to creating effective and safe herbal tablets. The quality of the herbs directly impacts the potency, efficacy, and safety of the final product. This section provides guidance on how to choose the best herbs for your herbal tablets, ensuring that they deliver the intended therapeutic benefits.

Understanding Herb Quality

The quality of herbs can vary significantly based on factors such as source, cultivation methods, and processing. Understanding these factors helps in selecting herbs that are both effective and safe.

- **Purity**: High-quality herbs should be free from contaminants such as pesticides, heavy metals, and microbial contaminants. Purity is crucial for ensuring that the herbs do not cause adverse effects and that their therapeutic properties are preserved.

- **Potency**: The potency of herbs refers to the concentration of active compounds that provide therapeutic effects. Potency can be influenced by the part of the plant used (roots, leaves, flowers), the growing conditions, and the processing methods.

- **Freshness**: Fresh herbs generally contain higher levels of active compounds compared to older or stale herbs. Freshness also affects the aroma, color, and overall quality of the herbs.

Sourcing High-Quality Herbs

Choosing reputable sources for your herbs ensures that you receive high-quality, reliable materials for your herbal tablets.

- **Certified Organic**: Opt for herbs that are certified organic, as this certification indicates that the herbs are grown without synthetic pesticides, herbicides, or genetically modified organisms (GMOs). Organic herbs are often preferred for their purity and environmental sustainability.

- **Reputable Suppliers**: Purchase herbs from well-established suppliers with a reputation for quality and transparency. Look for suppliers who provide information about their sourcing practices, quality control measures, and third-party testing results.

- **Wildcrafted Herbs**: Wildcrafted herbs are gathered from their natural habitats, often resulting in higher potency. Ensure that wildcrafted herbs are collected sustainably and ethically, with respect for the environment and local regulations.

Evaluating Herb Appearance and Smell

Visual and olfactory assessments can provide insights into the quality of herbs before purchase.

- **Color**: High-quality herbs should have vibrant and consistent colors. Dull or faded colors may indicate that the herbs are old or improperly stored.

- **Aroma**: Fresh herbs have a strong, characteristic aroma. If the herbs have a weak or off-putting smell, it may indicate that they are stale or contaminated.

- **Texture**: The texture of herbs can also indicate quality. For example, dried herbs should be crisp and break easily, while excessively brittle or powdery herbs may be too old.

Identifying Commonly Used Herbs

Familiarizing yourself with commonly used herbs and their specific qualities helps in making informed choices for your herbal tablets.

- **Echinacea**: Known for its immune-supportive properties, high-quality echinacea should have a strong, earthy aroma and be rich in active compounds such as echinacoside.

- **Ginger**: Valued for its digestive and anti-inflammatory benefits, fresh ginger should be firm with a spicy aroma. Dried ginger should be finely ground and free from clumps.

- **Turmeric**: This herb is celebrated for its anti-inflammatory and antioxidant properties. High-quality turmeric should have a deep orange color and a pungent aroma, indicating the presence of curcumin.

- **Valerian Root**: Used for its calming effects, valerian root should have a strong, characteristic smell and be free from mold or foreign materials.

Preparing Herbs for Tablets

Proper preparation of herbs ensures that their active compounds are effectively incorporated into the tablets.

- **Drying and Grinding**: Herbs should be dried properly to prevent mold growth and preserve their potency. Once dried, they can be ground into a fine powder using a grinder or mill.

- **Extracting**: For herbs that are not used in their raw form, extracts can be made using solvents such as alcohol or water. Ensure that extracts are concentrated and standardized for consistent potency.

- **Blending**: When combining multiple herbs, ensure that the blend is well-balanced and that each herb contributes its intended effects. Proper blending also ensures uniform distribution of active compounds in the tablets.

Testing and Quality Assurance

Quality assurance measures help confirm that the herbs used meet the required standards for safety and effectiveness.

- **Third-Party Testing**: Some suppliers provide third-party testing results that verify the quality and purity of their herbs. Look for certificates of analysis that indicate testing for contaminants, potency, and authenticity.

- **Organoleptic Evaluation**: Use organoleptic methods (sensory evaluation) to assess the appearance, aroma, and texture of herbs. This can help identify any issues with quality before use.

By following these guidelines for choosing high-quality herbs, you can ensure that your herbal tablets are effective, safe, and of the highest standard. Selecting and preparing the right ingredients is a crucial step in creating herbal remedies that deliver the desired therapeutic benefits.

Techniques for Making Herbal Tablets

Creating herbal tablets involves a series of precise steps to ensure that the final product is effective, safe, and consistent. This section outlines the key techniques involved in making herbal tablets, from preparing the herbal ingredients to pressing and quality control.

Preparing Herbal Ingredients

The preparation of herbal ingredients is crucial for the effectiveness of the tablets. Proper preparation ensures that the herbs are in the optimal form for tablet production.

- **Drying and Grinding Herbs**: Begin by drying the herbs thoroughly to prevent mold and degradation. Once dried, use a grinder or mill to convert the herbs into a fine powder. This powder should be uniform in texture to ensure even distribution in the tablets.

- **Creating Extracts**: For some herbs, making extracts can be beneficial. Extracts are concentrated forms of the herb's active compounds. Use solvents such as alcohol, vinegar, or water to create tinctures, decoctions, or infusions. Ensure the extracts are standardized to achieve consistent potency.

- **Combining Ingredients**: Mix the powdered herbs with any additional ingredients or excipients needed for tablet formation. Excipients, such as binders and fillers, help to bind the herbal powder and aid in the formation of tablets.

Formulating the Tablet Mixture

Formulating the mixture for tablet making involves blending herbs and excipients in precise proportions to ensure effectiveness and consistency.

- **Measuring Ingredients**: Use a digital scale to accurately measure the herbal powders and excipients. Proper measurement is crucial for ensuring that each tablet contains the correct dosage of active ingredients.

- **Blending**: Combine the powdered herbs and excipients in a mixing bowl or container. Use a spatula or mechanical mixer to ensure thorough blending. The goal is to achieve a uniform mixture where the herbs are evenly distributed.

- **Creating a Uniform Blend**: For larger batches, consider using a ribbon blender or other mixing equipment to ensure that the blend is consistent. This step is important to avoid variations in tablet potency.

Pressing the Tablets

The pressing process involves compressing the herbal powder mixture into solid tablet form. This step requires the appropriate equipment and techniques to ensure that the tablets are uniform and of high quality.

- **Using a Tablet Press**: A tablet press is a machine that compresses the herbal powder mixture into tablets. Adjust the press settings to achieve the desired tablet size and hardness. Ensure that the machine is clean and well-maintained to avoid contamination.

- **Manual Tablet Molds**: For small-scale production, manual tablet molds can be used. These molds are available in various shapes and sizes. Fill the molds with the herbal powder mixture and use a tamper to compress the powder firmly.

- **Checking Tablet Hardness**: After pressing, check the hardness of the tablets. Tablets should be firm but not excessively hard. Use a tablet hardness tester to ensure that the tablets meet quality standards for disintegration and dissolution.

Quality Control and Testing

Ensuring the quality of herbal tablets involves several quality control measures to verify that the tablets are effective, safe, and consistent.

- **Uniformity Testing**: Check for uniformity in tablet size, weight, and dosage. Use a caliper to measure tablet dimensions and a scale to weigh samples. Consistent size and weight are indicators of proper tablet formulation.

- **Disintegration Testing**: Test the tablets for disintegration to ensure that they dissolve properly in the digestive system. This can be done using a disintegration tester or by placing tablets in a controlled environment to observe their breakdown over time.

- **Stability Testing**: Evaluate the stability of the tablets over time to ensure that they retain their potency and effectiveness. Store samples under various conditions (e.g., different temperatures and humidity levels) and monitor for any changes in quality.

- **Microbial Testing**: Conduct microbial testing to check for contamination. This is especially important for tablets that will be stored for extended periods. Ensure that the tablets are free from harmful microorganisms.

Packaging and Storage

Proper packaging and storage are essential for maintaining the quality and longevity of herbal tablets.

- **Packaging**: Use airtight containers to protect the tablets from moisture, light, and air. Glass jars or high-quality plastic bottles with tight-sealing lids are recommended. Ensure that the packaging is clean and free from contaminants.

- **Labeling**: Clearly label the containers with information about the contents, dosage, and expiration date. Accurate labeling helps in proper usage and ensures that the tablets are used within their effective period.

- **Storage Conditions**: Store tablets in a cool, dry place away from direct sunlight and humidity. Proper storage conditions help preserve the potency and shelf life of the tablets.

By following these techniques for making herbal tablets, you can produce high-quality, effective, and safe herbal remedies. Each step, from preparation and formulation to pressing and quality control, contributes to the overall success of your herbal tablet production process.

Chapter 3: Herbal Tablet Formulations

Understanding Dosages and Potency

Proper understanding of dosages and potency is critical for creating effective and safe herbal tablets. This section explains the concepts of dosage and potency, how to calculate appropriate dosages, and how to ensure that your herbal tablets are both effective and safe for consumption.

What is Potency?

Potency refers to the strength or concentration of the active compounds in an herb that are responsible for its therapeutic effects. The potency of an herb can be influenced by various factors, including:

- **Part of the Plant Used**: Different parts of the plant (roots, leaves, flowers, seeds) contain varying concentrations of active compounds. For instance, the roots of certain herbs may have higher concentrations of therapeutic constituents compared to the leaves.

- **Growing Conditions**: The environment where the herb is cultivated, including soil quality, climate, and exposure to sunlight, can affect its potency. Herbs grown in optimal conditions generally have higher levels of active compounds.

- **Processing and Storage**: How the herb is processed and stored can impact its potency. Proper drying, grinding, and storage methods help preserve the active compounds.

Determining Dosages

Determining the correct dosage for herbal tablets involves calculating the amount of active ingredients required to achieve the desired therapeutic effect. This can be challenging due to variations in herb potency and individual patient needs.

- **Standard Dosages**: Many herbs have established standard dosages based on clinical studies and traditional use. These dosages provide a starting point for formulating your tablets. Always refer to reputable sources or consult with a healthcare professional for guidance.

- **Active Compound Content**: Calculate the amount of active compound needed per tablet based on the desired dosage. This involves understanding the concentration of active compounds in the herbal powder or extract. For example, if a herb contains 5% active compound and the target dose is 100 mg, you would need 2 grams of the herb powder to achieve the required dosage.

- **Individual Factors**: Consider individual factors such as age, weight, and health conditions when determining dosages. Dosage adjustments may be necessary to tailor the formulation to specific needs.

Calculating Dosages for Tablets

Accurate dosage calculation ensures that each tablet delivers a consistent amount of active ingredients. Here's a step-by-step guide to calculating dosages for herbal tablets:

- **Determine the Target Dosage**: Identify the recommended dosage of the active ingredient per tablet. For instance, if the target dosage is 200 mg of a particular herb per tablet, use this as a reference.

- **Measure Active Ingredient Concentration**: Assess the concentration of the active ingredient in the herbal powder or extract. For example, if the herb powder contains 10% active compound, then 1 gram of the powder provides 100 mg of the active ingredient.

- **Calculate Required Herb Powder**: Based on the active ingredient concentration, calculate the amount of herb powder needed. Using the previous example, if you need 200 mg of active ingredient per tablet and the powder contains 10% active compound, you would need 2 grams of herb powder per tablet.

- **Incorporate Excipients**: Factor in the amount of excipients required to create the tablet. Excipients help with tablet formation and stability but do not contribute to the therapeutic effects.

Testing and Ensuring Potency

Testing and quality control are essential to ensure that your herbal tablets have the intended potency and effectiveness.

- **Potency Testing**: Conduct laboratory tests to verify the concentration of active compounds in your herbal tablets. High-performance liquid chromatography (HPLC) and other analytical methods can be used to measure potency.

- **Consistency Checks**: Regularly test tablet batches to ensure consistency in dosage and potency. Monitor for any variations and adjust formulations as needed.

- **Stability Testing**: Perform stability tests to assess how the potency of the tablets changes over time. Store samples under different conditions and evaluate their potency at various intervals.

Adjusting Dosages

Adjusting dosages may be necessary based on feedback from users or changes in the formulation.

- **User Feedback**: Collect feedback from users regarding the effectiveness and any side effects of the herbal tablets. Adjust dosages if needed to enhance efficacy or reduce adverse effects.

- **Formulation Changes**: If you modify the formulation by adding or removing ingredients, recalculate the dosages and reassess the potency to ensure that the tablets remain effective.

Safety Considerations

Ensuring the safety of herbal tablets involves careful consideration of dosages and potential interactions.

- **Avoiding Overdose**: Be mindful of the potential for overdose, especially with potent herbs. Adhere to recommended dosages and avoid excessive use.

- **Herb Interactions**: Be aware of possible interactions between herbs and other medications or supplements. Ensure that the herbal tablets do not interfere with conventional treatments or cause adverse effects.

- **Consulting Professionals**: For complex formulations or specific health conditions, consult with healthcare professionals or herbalists to ensure that the dosages and potency are appropriate.

Understanding and managing dosages and potency are key to creating effective herbal tablets that provide consistent and beneficial therapeutic effects. By following these guidelines, you can ensure that your herbal tablets are safe, effective, and reliable for users.

Binding Agents and Preservation

The selection of binding agents and preservation methods is essential for creating high-quality herbal tablets that are both effective and durable. This section explores the role of binding agents in tablet formation and the various preservation techniques to maintain the stability and shelf life of your herbal tablets.

Binding Agents

Binding agents are substances used to hold the herbal powder together and ensure the formation of a solid, cohesive tablet. They help in creating tablets with the right hardness and disintegration properties.

- **Types of Binding Agents**:

- Cellulose-Based Binders: Common binders such as microcrystalline cellulose (MCC) and hydroxypropyl methylcellulose (HPMC) are derived from plant fibers. They help in forming a stable tablet matrix and are widely used due to their effectiveness and safety.

- Starch-Based Binders: Starch and its derivatives (e.g., pregelatinized starch) are used as binders and disintegrants. They provide good binding properties and help tablets break down properly in the digestive system.

- Gums: Natural gums such as guar gum, xanthan gum, and acacia gum can be used as binding agents. They form a gel-like consistency when mixed with water, aiding in tablet cohesion.

- Synthetic Polymers: Synthetic binders like polyvinylpyrrolidone (PVP) and polyethylene glycol (PEG) are used for their strong binding properties and ability to enhance tablet stability.

- **Choosing the Right Binder**: Select a binder based on the desired tablet hardness, disintegration time, and compatibility with the herbal ingredients. For instance, cellulose-based binders are ideal for herbal tablets that require a strong and durable matrix.

- **Incorporating Binders**: Binders are usually mixed with the herbal powder and other excipients in the formulation process. The amount of binder needed depends on the specific formulation and the desired properties of the final tablet.

Preservation Techniques

Preservation techniques are crucial for maintaining the quality, potency, and shelf life of herbal tablets. Proper preservation prevents degradation of active ingredients and protects tablets from environmental factors.

- **Moisture Control**:

  - **Desiccants**: Use desiccants like silica gel or activated clay to absorb moisture and prevent tablet degradation. Place desiccants in the packaging to keep the tablets dry.

  - **Humidity Control**: Store tablets in environments with controlled humidity levels to prevent moisture absorption, which can lead to tablet caking or degradation.

- **Temperature Management**:

- **Cool Storage**: Store tablets in a cool, dry place away from direct sunlight and high temperatures. Excessive heat can cause the herbal components to break down and lose potency.

- **Refrigeration**: For certain formulations, refrigeration may be necessary to maintain stability. Ensure that the tablets are well-packaged to avoid moisture accumulation.

- **Light Protection**:

  - **Opaque Packaging**: Use opaque or dark-colored containers to protect tablets from light exposure, which can degrade sensitive herbal compounds.

  - **Light-Blocking Materials**: Employ packaging materials that block UV light to further safeguard the tablets.

- **Packaging Materials**:

  - **Airtight Containers**: Use airtight containers such as glass jars or high-quality plastic bottles with secure lids. Airtight packaging helps protect the tablets from air exposure, which can lead to oxidation and loss of potency.

- **Blister Packs**: For added protection, consider using blister packs that provide individual compartments for each tablet. This packaging helps prevent moisture and contamination.

- **Preservative Additives**:

  - **Natural Preservatives**: Some natural preservatives, such as vitamin E or rosemary extract, can be added to the formulation to extend shelf life. These additives help inhibit oxidation and microbial growth.

  - **Chemical Preservatives**: In some cases, chemical preservatives may be used, but they should be selected based on safety and regulatory guidelines.

Quality Control and Testing

Ensuring the effectiveness of binding agents and preservation methods requires regular quality control and testing:

- **Tablet Hardness Testing**: Measure the hardness of the tablets to ensure that they are neither too soft nor too hard. Proper hardness ensures that the tablets maintain their shape during handling and consumption.

- **Disintegration Testing**: Test the disintegration time of the tablets to confirm that they break down appropriately in the digestive system. This ensures that the active ingredients are released and absorbed effectively.

- **Stability Testing**: Conduct stability tests to evaluate how the tablets fare under various storage conditions over time. Monitor for changes in potency, appearance, and disintegration.

Practical Tips for Binding and Preservation

- **Consistency in Binder Use**: Use consistent amounts of binder across batches to maintain uniform tablet quality. Adjust binder levels based on formulation needs and tablet properties.

- **Regular Monitoring**: Regularly check the condition of stored tablets and packaging materials. Replace or repackage tablets if any signs of degradation or moisture are observed.

- **Compliance with Regulations**: Follow relevant regulations and guidelines for the use of binders and preservatives. Ensure that all materials used are safe and approved for herbal tablet production.

By understanding and applying the principles of binding agents and preservation techniques, you can produce high-quality herbal tablets that maintain their effectiveness and shelf life. Proper formulation, storage, and quality control are key to ensuring the success of your herbal tablet products.

Storage and Shelf Life

Proper storage and management of shelf life are critical to ensuring that herbal tablets remain effective, safe, and stable throughout their intended use. This section provides comprehensive guidelines on how to store herbal tablets and how to manage their shelf life.

Importance of Proper Storage

Effective storage practices help maintain the potency and quality of herbal tablets by protecting them from environmental factors that can lead to degradation. Proper storage is essential for preserving the active ingredients and extending the shelf life of the tablets.

- **Temperature**: Store herbal tablets in a cool environment to prevent heat-induced degradation. Excessive heat can cause the active compounds to break down, leading to reduced efficacy. Ideally, tablets should be kept at a temperature below 25°C (77°F).

- **Humidity**: Control humidity levels to prevent moisture absorption, which can lead to mold growth, caking, or premature degradation. Tablets should be stored in a dry place with low humidity. Using desiccants in the packaging can help maintain a dry environment.

- **Light**: Protect tablets from direct sunlight and UV light, which can cause chemical reactions that degrade active ingredients. Use opaque or dark-colored containers to shield the tablets from light exposure.

- **Air Exposure**: Minimize exposure to air to prevent oxidation of active compounds. Airtight containers or blister packs are ideal for maintaining a controlled environment and protecting tablets from air.

Storage Solutions

Selecting appropriate storage solutions is crucial for maintaining the quality of herbal tablets. Here are some effective storage methods:

- **Airtight Containers**: Use airtight containers made of glass or high-quality plastic to keep moisture and air out. Ensure that the lids are securely fastened to maintain the integrity of the tablets.

- **Blister Packs**: Blister packs are excellent for single-dose protection, preventing exposure to moisture and air. Each tablet is individually sealed, which helps preserve freshness and potency.

- **Vacuum Sealing**: Vacuum sealing removes air from the packaging, reducing oxidation and extending shelf life. This method is effective for bulk storage but requires specialized equipment.

- **Refrigeration**: For certain formulations or long-term storage, refrigeration may be necessary. Ensure that the tablets are well-sealed and protected from moisture when stored in the refrigerator.

Managing Shelf Life

Shelf life refers to the period during which herbal tablets remain effective and safe for consumption. Managing shelf life involves monitoring, labeling, and adhering to expiration dates.

- **Expiration Dates**: Assign expiration dates based on stability testing and the expected shelf life of the tablets. This information should be clearly labeled on the packaging to inform users of the recommended usage period.

- **Stability Testing**: Conduct stability tests to determine how long the tablets maintain their potency and quality under various storage conditions. Regularly evaluate the tablets for changes in appearance, potency, and efficacy.

- **Batch Tracking**: Implement batch tracking systems to monitor the production and expiration dates of each batch. This allows for effective management of inventory and ensures that outdated tablets are removed from circulation.

- **Handling and Distribution**: Ensure that tablets are handled properly during distribution and storage to prevent damage. Train staff on best practices for handling, storing, and shipping herbal tablets.

Quality Control

Regular quality control checks are essential for ensuring that herbal tablets remain within their specified shelf life and maintain their intended quality.

- **Visual Inspection**: Inspect tablets for any signs of physical degradation, such as discoloration, crumbling, or mold growth. Any abnormalities should be addressed immediately.

- **Potency Testing**: Periodically test the potency of the tablets to ensure that they contain the correct amount of active ingredients. This helps verify that the tablets remain effective throughout their shelf life.

- **Environmental Monitoring**: Monitor storage conditions such as temperature, humidity, and light exposure to ensure that they remain within the recommended ranges. Adjust storage practices as needed to maintain optimal conditions.

Best Practices for Consumers

Educating consumers on proper storage practices can help extend the shelf life of herbal tablets and ensure their effectiveness.

- **Storage Instructions**: Provide clear storage instructions on the packaging, including recommendations for temperature, humidity, and light protection.

- **Usage Guidance**: Advise consumers to use tablets before the expiration date and to follow any specific storage guidelines provided.

- **Return and Disposal**: Encourage consumers to return expired or damaged tablets for proper disposal and replacement, if applicable.

By adhering to proper storage practices and managing shelf life effectively, you can ensure that your herbal tablets remain potent, safe, and of high quality throughout their intended use. Implementing these guidelines helps maintain the efficacy and integrity of your products, providing reliable natural remedies for users.

Chapter 4: Remedy Recipes for Common Health Issues

Immune System Support

Echinacea and Elderberry Tablets

Echinacea and elderberry are two of the most popular herbs used to support immune health. Combining these powerful herbs into tablet form provides a convenient way to harness their benefits. This section covers the benefits, ingredients, and preparation process for making effective echinacea and elderberry tablets.

Benefits of Echinacea and Elderberry

- **Echinacea**: Echinacea is well-known for its immune-boosting properties. It helps stimulate the body's natural defenses, making it a popular choice for preventing and treating colds and infections. Echinacea is also thought to reduce inflammation and promote overall well-being.

- **Elderberry**: Elderberry is rich in antioxidants and has been traditionally used to combat respiratory infections, such as colds and flu. It is known for its antiviral properties and can help reduce the severity and duration of illness. Elderberries are also beneficial for their immune-supportive effects.

Ingredients

- **Echinacea Root Powder**: Known for its immune-stimulating effects.

- **Elderberry Powder**: Provides antioxidant support and helps with respiratory health.

- **Vitamin C Powder**: Enhances immune function and supports overall health.

- **Binder**: Such as cellulose powder or starch, to help form the tablets.

Preparation Process

1. **Gather Ingredients**:

   o **Echinacea Root Powder**: 30%

   o **Elderberry Powder**: 30%

   o **Vitamin C Powder**: 10%

   o **Binder**: 30% (such as cellulose powder)

2. **Mixing**:

- In a clean, dry bowl, combine the echinacea root powder, elderberry powder, and vitamin C powder. Mix thoroughly to ensure an even distribution of all ingredients.

- Gradually add the binder to the mixture. The binder helps hold the tablet together and ensures proper consistency.

3. **Forming Tablets**:

- Using a tablet press or a manual tablet-making tool, compress the mixture into tablets. Ensure that each tablet is uniformly sized and well-compressed to avoid crumbling.

- If you don't have a tablet press, you can also use a mortar and pestle to blend and compress the mixture manually, although this may be less efficient.

4. **Drying**:

- Allow the tablets to dry completely before storing them. This helps prevent moisture from causing the tablets to degrade. Place them on a clean, dry surface and let them air dry for several hours or as recommended by your tablet press instructions.

5. **Storage**:

- Store the dried tablets in airtight containers to protect them from moisture, light, and air. Keep the containers in a cool, dry place to maintain the potency and shelf life of the tablets.

- Label the containers with the date of preparation and any other relevant information.

Dosage and Usage

- **Recommended Dosage**: Follow the recommended dosage instructions based on the potency of the tablets and individual health needs. Typically, 1-2 tablets per day may be sufficient, but consult with a healthcare provider for personalized advice.

- **Usage Instructions**: Take the tablets with a glass of water, ideally between meals. Consistent use can help support immune function and overall health.

Quality Control

- **Check for Uniformity**: Ensure that tablets are of uniform size and weight for consistent dosing. Inspect tablets for any signs of physical degradation, such as cracks or discoloration.

- **Potency Testing**: Periodically test the potency of the tablets to ensure they contain the intended levels of active ingredients.

Conclusion

Echinacea and elderberry tablets offer a natural and convenient way to support immune health. By following the preparation process and storage guidelines, you can create effective herbal tablets that help bolster the body's defenses and promote overall wellness.

Astragalus and Ginger Tablets

Astragalus and ginger are renowned for their supportive effects on immune health and overall vitality. Combining these two herbs into tablet form offers a powerful remedy for enhancing immune function and promoting general wellness. This section provides a comprehensive guide to creating effective astragalus and ginger tablets.

Benefits of Astragalus and Ginger

- **Astragalus Root**: Astragalus is a traditional Chinese herb known for its immune-boosting and adaptogenic properties. It helps strengthen the immune system, increase energy levels, and support the body's natural defense mechanisms. Astragalus is also beneficial for its anti-inflammatory and antioxidant effects.

- **Ginger Root**: Ginger is well-known for its digestive and anti-inflammatory benefits. It helps improve circulation, reduce nausea, and supports overall immune health. Ginger also has antioxidant properties and can aid in reducing inflammation and boosting overall vitality.

Ingredients

- **Astragalus Root Powder**: Known for its immune-enhancing and adaptogenic effects.

- **Ginger Root Powder**: Provides digestive support and anti-inflammatory benefits.

- **Binder**: Such as cellulose powder or starch, to facilitate tablet formation.

- **Optional Additives**: Such as stevia or other natural sweeteners, if desired for taste.

Preparation Process

1. **Gather Ingredients**:

   o **Astragalus Root Powder**: 40%

- **Ginger Root Powder**: 40%

- **Binder**: 20% (such as cellulose powder)

2. **Mixing**:

   - In a clean, dry bowl, combine the astragalus root powder and ginger root powder. Mix thoroughly to ensure an even distribution of both herbs.

   - Gradually incorporate the binder into the mixture. The binder helps the herbs adhere together and ensures the tablets hold their shape.

3. **Forming Tablets**:

   - Using a tablet press or a manual tablet-making tool, compress the mixture into tablets. Ensure that each tablet is uniformly sized and well-compressed to prevent breakage.

   - If a tablet press is not available, you can use a mortar and pestle to mix and compress the herbs manually, though this method may be less precise.

4. **Drying**:

- Allow the tablets to air dry completely before storing them. Proper drying helps prevent moisture from causing the tablets to degrade. Place them on a clean, dry surface and let them dry for several hours or as per the tablet press instructions.

5. **Storage**:

   - Store the dried tablets in airtight containers to protect them from moisture, light, and air. Keep the containers in a cool, dry place to maintain the tablets' potency and shelf life.

   - Label the containers with the preparation date and any relevant information for easy reference.

Dosage and Usage

- **Recommended Dosage**: Typically, 1-2 tablets per day are sufficient, but dosage may vary based on individual needs and the potency of the tablets. Consult with a healthcare provider for personalized recommendations.

- **Usage Instructions**: Take the tablets with a glass of water, preferably between meals. Regular use can help enhance immune function and support overall health.

Quality Control

- **Check for Uniformity**: Ensure that the tablets are of consistent size and weight for accurate dosing. Inspect the tablets for any signs of physical damage or degradation.

- **Potency Testing**: Periodically test the potency of the tablets to ensure they contain the intended amounts of active ingredients.

Conclusion

Astragalus and ginger tablets provide a convenient and effective way to support immune health and overall vitality. By following the preparation and storage guidelines, you can create high-quality herbal tablets that harness the benefits of these powerful herbs, helping to enhance well-being and support a healthy immune system.

Andrographis and Garlic Tablets

Andrographis and garlic are celebrated for their potent health benefits, particularly in supporting immune function and combating infections. Combining these herbs into tablet form offers a powerful remedy for enhancing overall health and well-being. This section provides a detailed guide for preparing effective andrographis and garlic tablets.

Benefits of Andrographis and Garlic

- **Andrographis**: Known as a traditional remedy in Ayurveda and Chinese medicine, andrographis is renowned for its immune-boosting and anti-inflammatory properties. It helps strengthen the immune system, alleviate symptoms of respiratory infections, and reduce inflammation throughout the body.

- **Garlic**: Garlic is widely recognized for its antimicrobial and immune-enhancing effects. It contains allicin, a compound with potent antibacterial, antiviral, and antifungal properties. Garlic supports cardiovascular health, reduces inflammation, and boosts the immune system's ability to fend off infections.

Ingredients

- **Andrographis Powder**: Provides immune support and anti-inflammatory benefits.

- **Garlic Powder**: Known for its antimicrobial and immune-boosting properties.

- **Binder**: Such as cellulose powder or starch, to ensure tablet cohesion.

- **Optional Additives**: Such as stevia or natural flavorings, if desired.

Preparation Process

1. **Gather Ingredients**:

   ○ **Andrographis Powder**: 50%

   ○ **Garlic Powder**: 40%

   ○ **Binder**: 10% (such as cellulose powder)

2. **Mixing**:

   ○ In a clean, dry bowl, combine the andrographis powder and garlic powder. Stir thoroughly to ensure an even distribution of both powders.

   ○ Gradually add the binder to the mixture. The binder helps the herbs adhere together and ensures that the tablets maintain their shape.

3. **Forming Tablets**:

   ○ Using a tablet press or a manual tablet-making tool, compress the mixture into tablets. Ensure each tablet is uniformly sized and well-compressed to avoid crumbling.

o If you don't have a tablet press, you can manually mix and compress the ingredients using a mortar and pestle, though this method may be less precise.

4. **Drying**:

   o Allow the tablets to air dry completely before storing. Proper drying prevents moisture from causing the tablets to break down. Place them on a clean, dry surface and let them dry for several hours or according to the tablet press instructions.

5. **Storage**:

   o Store the dried tablets in airtight containers to protect them from moisture, light, and air. Keep the containers in a cool, dry place to maintain the tablets' potency and shelf life.

   o Label the containers with the preparation date and any relevant information.

Dosage and Usage

- **Recommended Dosage**: Typically, 1-2 tablets per day are sufficient, but dosage can vary based on the tablets' potency and individual health needs. Consult with a healthcare provider for personalized dosage recommendations.

- **Usage Instructions**: Take the tablets with a glass of water, preferably between meals. Regular use can help support immune health and overall well-being.

Quality Control

- **Check for Uniformity**: Ensure the tablets are of consistent size and weight for accurate dosing. Inspect the tablets for any signs of damage or physical degradation.

- **Potency Testing**: Periodically test the potency of the tablets to ensure they contain the intended levels of active ingredients.

Conclusion

Andrographis and garlic tablets offer a convenient and effective way to enhance immune function and support overall health. By following the preparation and storage guidelines, you can create high-quality herbal tablets that leverage the powerful benefits of these herbs, promoting well-being and resilience against infections.

Reishi Mushroom and Shiitake Tablets

Reishi and shiitake mushrooms are highly regarded in traditional medicine for their immune-enhancing and health-promoting properties. Combining these mushrooms into tablet form provides a convenient way to enjoy their benefits. This section details the preparation of effective reishi mushroom and shiitake tablets.

Benefits of Reishi and Shiitake

- **Reishi Mushroom**: Often referred to as the "mushroom of immortality," reishi is celebrated for its immune-boosting, anti-inflammatory, and adaptogenic properties. It helps enhance immune function, reduce stress, and support overall vitality. Reishi is also known for its potential to improve sleep quality and support heart health.

- **Shiitake Mushroom**: Shiitake mushrooms are valued for their immune-supporting and antimicrobial properties. They contain compounds such as lentinans and eritadenines, which help strengthen the immune system and support cardiovascular health. Shiitake mushrooms are also rich in vitamins and minerals that promote overall health.

Ingredients

- **Reishi Mushroom Powder**: Provides immune support and adaptogenic benefits.

- **Shiitake Mushroom Powder**: Offers immune-enhancing and cardiovascular support.

- **Binder**: Such as cellulose powder or starch, to help form the tablets.

- **Optional Additives**: Such as a natural flavoring or sweetener if desired.

Preparation Process

1. **Gather Ingredients**:

   - **Reishi Mushroom Powder**: 50%

   - **Shiitake Mushroom Powder**: 40%

   - **Binder**: 10% (such as cellulose powder or starch)

2. **Mixing**:

   - In a clean, dry bowl, combine the reishi mushroom powder and shiitake mushroom powder. Stir well to ensure even distribution of both powders.

- Gradually add the binder to the mixture. The binder helps the ingredients adhere together and ensures that the tablets maintain their shape and integrity.

3. **Forming Tablets**:

- Use a tablet press or manual tablet-making tool to compress the mixture into tablets. Ensure that each tablet is uniformly sized and well-compressed to prevent crumbling.

- If you do not have a tablet press, you can use a mortar and pestle to blend and compress the ingredients manually, although this method may be less precise.

4. **Drying**:

- Allow the tablets to air dry completely before storing them. Proper drying is essential to prevent moisture from causing the tablets to degrade. Place them on a clean, dry surface and let them dry for several hours or according to the tablet press instructions.

5. **Storage**:

- Store the dried tablets in airtight containers to protect them from moisture, light, and air. Keep the containers in a cool, dry place to maintain the tablets' potency and shelf life.

- Label the containers with the preparation date and any relevant information.

Dosage and Usage

- **Recommended Dosage**: Generally, 1-2 tablets per day are adequate, but dosage may vary based on the tablets' potency and individual health needs. Consult with a healthcare provider for personalized recommendations.

- **Usage Instructions**: Take the tablets with a glass of water, preferably between meals. Consistent use can help support immune function and overall health.

Quality Control

- **Check for Uniformity**: Ensure that the tablets are of consistent size and weight for accurate dosing. Inspect the tablets for any signs of physical damage or degradation.

- **Potency Testing**: Periodically test the potency of the tablets to confirm that they contain the intended levels of active ingredients.

Conclusion

Reishi mushroom and shiitake tablets offer a convenient and effective way to harness the health benefits of these powerful mushrooms. By following the preparation and storage guidelines, you can create high-quality herbal tablets that support immune health, vitality, and overall well-being.

Digestive Health

Peppermint and Ginger Tablets

Peppermint and ginger are both renowned for their digestive and soothing properties. Combining these two herbs into tablet form offers a powerful remedy for alleviating digestive discomfort, reducing nausea, and promoting overall digestive health. This section provides a comprehensive guide to preparing effective peppermint and ginger tablets.

Benefits of Peppermint and Ginger

- **Peppermint**: Peppermint is well-known for its ability to relieve digestive issues such as bloating, gas, and indigestion. It helps relax the muscles of the gastrointestinal tract, reducing symptoms of discomfort.

Peppermint also has a calming effect on the digestive system and can help alleviate nausea.

- **Ginger**: Ginger is widely used for its anti-nausea and digestive benefits. It helps stimulate digestion, reduce inflammation, and alleviate nausea. Ginger also supports healthy gastric motility, which can be beneficial for individuals experiencing digestive issues like indigestion or bloating.

Ingredients

- **Peppermint Leaf Powder**: Provides relief from digestive discomfort and supports healthy digestion.

- **Ginger Root Powder**: Aids in digestion, reduces nausea, and supports overall digestive health.

- **Binder**: Such as cellulose powder or starch, to ensure proper tablet formation.

- **Optional Additives**: Natural flavorings or sweeteners, if desired, to enhance taste.

Preparation Process

1. **Gather Ingredients**:

   o **Peppermint Leaf Powder**: 50%

- **Ginger Root Powder**: 40%

- **Binder**: 10% (such as cellulose powder or starch)

2. **Mixing**:

   - In a clean, dry bowl, combine the peppermint leaf powder and ginger root powder. Mix thoroughly to ensure an even distribution of both powders.

   - Gradually add the binder to the mixture. The binder helps the ingredients adhere together and ensures that the tablets maintain their shape.

3. **Forming Tablets**:

   - Using a tablet press or manual tablet-making tool, compress the mixture into tablets. Ensure each tablet is uniformly sized and well-compressed to avoid crumbling.

   - If a tablet press is not available, you can use a mortar and pestle to mix and compress the ingredients manually, though this method may be less precise.

4. **Drying**:

o Allow the tablets to air dry completely before storing them. Proper drying is essential to prevent moisture from causing the tablets to break down. Place them on a clean, dry surface and let them dry for several hours or according to the tablet press instructions.

5. **Storage**:

   o Store the dried tablets in airtight containers to protect them from moisture, light, and air. Keep the containers in a cool, dry place to maintain the tablets' potency and shelf life.

   o Label the containers with the preparation date and any relevant information.

Dosage and Usage

• **Recommended Dosage**: Typically, 1-2 tablets per day are sufficient for supporting digestive health, but dosage may vary based on the tablets' potency and individual needs. Consult with a healthcare provider for personalized recommendations.

- **Usage Instructions**: Take the tablets with a glass of water, preferably between meals. Regular use can help support healthy digestion and alleviate digestive discomfort.

Quality Control

- **Check for Uniformity**: Ensure the tablets are of consistent size and weight for accurate dosing. Inspect the tablets for any signs of physical damage or degradation.

- **Potency Testing**: Periodically test the potency of the tablets to confirm they contain the intended levels of active ingredients.

Conclusion

Peppermint and ginger tablets offer a convenient and effective way to support digestive health and alleviate discomfort. By following the preparation and storage guidelines, you can create high-quality herbal tablets that harness the soothing benefits of peppermint and the digestive support of ginger, helping to maintain overall digestive wellness.

Dandelion and Licorice Root Tablets

Dandelion and licorice root are two powerful herbs known for their supportive roles in liver health, digestion, and overall well-being. Combining these herbs into tablet form offers a convenient way to harness their benefits for a range of health issues. This section provides a step-by-step guide to creating effective dandelion and licorice root tablets.

Benefits of Dandelion and Licorice Root

- **Dandelion**: Dandelion is a versatile herb with potent detoxifying and digestive properties. It supports liver health by promoting bile production and improving liver function. Dandelion also acts as a diuretic, helping to reduce water retention and support kidney health. Additionally, it has anti-inflammatory properties that can benefit overall wellness.

- **Licorice Root**: Licorice root is renowned for its soothing effects on the digestive system. It helps reduce inflammation and supports the mucosal lining of the stomach and intestines, making it useful for conditions like gastritis and ulcers. Licorice root also has liver-protective properties and can aid in balancing adrenal function.

Ingredients

- **Dandelion Root Powder**: Provides liver support, detoxification, and digestive benefits.

- **Licorice Root Powder**: Soothes the digestive tract, reduces inflammation, and supports liver health.

- **Binder**: Such as cellulose powder or starch, to ensure proper tablet formation.

- **Optional Additives**: Natural flavorings or sweeteners, if desired, to enhance taste.

Preparation Process

1. **Gather Ingredients**:

   o **Dandelion Root Powder**: 50%

   o **Licorice Root Powder**: 40%

   o **Binder**: 10% (such as cellulose powder or starch)

2. **Mixing**:

   o In a clean, dry bowl, combine the dandelion root powder and licorice root powder. Stir thoroughly to ensure even distribution of both powders.

o   Gradually add the binder to the mixture. The binder helps the herbs adhere together and ensures that the tablets hold their shape and consistency.

3. **Forming Tablets**:

o   Use a tablet press or manual tablet-making tool to compress the mixture into tablets. Ensure each tablet is uniformly sized and well-compressed to avoid crumbling.

o   If a tablet press is not available, you can use a mortar and pestle to blend and compress the ingredients manually, though this method may be less precise.

4. **Drying**:

o   Allow the tablets to air dry completely before storing them. Proper drying prevents moisture from causing the tablets to degrade. Place them on a clean, dry surface and let them dry for several hours or according to the tablet press instructions.

5. **Storage**:

- Store the dried tablets in airtight containers to protect them from moisture, light, and air. Keep the containers in a cool, dry place to maintain the tablets' potency and shelf life.

- Label the containers with the preparation date and any relevant information.

Dosage and Usage

- **Recommended Dosage**: Typically, 1-2 tablets per day are sufficient for supporting digestive and liver health, but dosage may vary based on the tablets' potency and individual needs. Consult with a healthcare provider for personalized dosage recommendations.

- **Usage Instructions**: Take the tablets with a glass of water, preferably between meals. Regular use can support liver function, aid digestion, and help reduce inflammation.

Quality Control

- **Check for Uniformity**: Ensure that the tablets are of consistent size and weight for accurate dosing. Inspect the tablets for any signs of physical damage or degradation.

- **Potency Testing**: Periodically test the potency of the tablets to confirm they contain the intended levels of active ingredients.

Conclusion

Dandelion and licorice root tablets offer a natural and effective way to support liver health, improve digestion, and reduce inflammation. By following the preparation and storage guidelines, you can create high-quality herbal tablets that leverage the therapeutic benefits of these herbs, promoting overall well-being and digestive health.

Fennel and Slippery Elm Tablets

Fennel and slippery elm are valued for their soothing and supportive properties for the digestive system. Combining these herbs into tablet form provides a convenient way to utilize their benefits for alleviating digestive discomfort, supporting gastrointestinal health, and promoting overall well-being. This section outlines the preparation of fennel and slippery elm tablets.

Benefits of Fennel and Slippery Elm

- **Fennel**: Fennel seeds are known for their carminative properties, which help relieve gas, bloating, and digestive discomfort. They support digestive health by relaxing the gastrointestinal tract and aiding in the elimination of gas. Fennel also has anti-inflammatory properties that can help soothe the digestive system.

- **Slippery Elm**: Slippery elm is prized for its mucilaginous properties, which help soothe and protect the mucosal lining of the gastrointestinal tract. It can be beneficial for conditions such as gastritis, ulcers, and inflammatory bowel diseases. Slippery elm also supports healthy digestion by improving nutrient absorption and reducing irritation.

Ingredients

- **Fennel Seed Powder**: Provides relief from gas, bloating, and supports overall digestive health.

- **Slippery Elm Bark Powder**: Soothes and protects the mucosal lining of the digestive tract, reduces inflammation.

- **Binder**: Such as cellulose powder or starch, to ensure proper tablet formation.

- **Optional Additives**: Natural flavorings or sweeteners, if desired, to enhance taste.

Preparation Process

1. **Gather Ingredients**:

- **Fennel Seed Powder**: 50%

- **Slippery Elm Bark Powder**: 40%

- **Binder**: 10% (such as cellulose powder or starch)

2. **Mixing**:

   - In a clean, dry bowl, combine the fennel seed powder and slippery elm bark powder. Stir thoroughly to ensure even distribution of both powders.

   - Gradually add the binder to the mixture. The binder helps the herbs adhere together and ensures that the tablets hold their shape and consistency.

3. **Forming Tablets**:

   - Use a tablet press or manual tablet-making tool to compress the mixture into tablets. Ensure that each tablet is uniformly sized and well-compressed to avoid crumbling.

   - If a tablet press is not available, you can use a mortar and pestle to blend and compress the ingredients manually, though this method may be less efficient.

4. **Drying**:

- Allow the tablets to air dry completely before storing them. Proper drying prevents moisture from causing the tablets to degrade. Place them on a clean, dry surface and let them dry for several hours or according to the tablet press instructions.

5. **Storage**:

   - Store the dried tablets in airtight containers to protect them from moisture, light, and air. Keep the containers in a cool, dry place to maintain the tablets' potency and shelf life.

   - Label the containers with the preparation date and any relevant information.

Dosage and Usage

- **Recommended Dosage**: Typically, 1-2 tablets per day are sufficient for supporting digestive health, but dosage may vary based on the tablets' potency and individual needs. Consult with a healthcare provider for personalized dosage recommendations.

- **Usage Instructions**: Take the tablets with a glass of water, preferably between meals. Regular use can help alleviate digestive discomfort, reduce bloating, and support overall gastrointestinal health.

Quality Control

- **Check for Uniformity**: Ensure that the tablets are of consistent size and weight for accurate dosing. Inspect the tablets for any signs of physical damage or degradation.

- **Potency Testing**: Periodically test the potency of the tablets to confirm they contain the intended levels of active ingredients.

Conclusion

Fennel and slippery elm tablets offer a natural and effective solution for supporting digestive health and soothing the gastrointestinal tract. By following the preparation and storage guidelines, you can create high-quality herbal tablets that leverage the therapeutic benefits of these herbs, helping to promote overall well-being and digestive comfort.

Marshmallow Root and Caraway Tablets

Marshmallow root and caraway are both known for their beneficial effects on the digestive system. Combining these herbs into tablet form creates a convenient remedy that can support digestive health, soothe inflammation, and alleviate discomfort. This section provides a comprehensive guide to preparing effective marshmallow root and caraway tablets.

Benefits of Marshmallow Root and Caraway

- **Marshmallow Root**: Marshmallow root is renowned for its mucilaginous properties, which help soothe and protect the mucosal lining of the digestive tract. It is beneficial for conditions such as gastritis, ulcers, and inflammatory bowel diseases. Marshmallow root helps to alleviate irritation, promote healing, and improve overall digestive comfort.

- **Caraway**: Caraway seeds are valued for their digestive benefits, including the relief of bloating, gas, and indigestion. Caraway promotes healthy digestion by relaxing the gastrointestinal tract and improving the breakdown and absorption of nutrients. It also has antimicrobial properties that support overall gut health.

Ingredients

- **Marshmallow Root Powder**: Provides soothing and protective benefits for the mucosal lining of the digestive tract.

- **Caraway Seed Powder**: Supports digestion, reduces bloating, and alleviates gas and indigestion.

- **Binder**: Such as cellulose powder or starch, to ensure proper tablet formation.

- **Optional Additives**: Natural flavorings or sweeteners, if desired, to enhance taste.

Preparation Process

1. **Gather Ingredients**:

   o **Marshmallow Root Powder**: 50%

   o **Caraway Seed Powder**: 40%

   o **Binder**: 10% (such as cellulose powder or starch)

2. **Mixing**:

   o In a clean, dry bowl, combine the marshmallow root powder and caraway seed powder. Stir thoroughly to ensure an even distribution of both powders.

   o Gradually add the binder to the mixture. The binder helps the herbs adhere together and ensures that the tablets maintain their shape and consistency.

3. **Forming Tablets**:

- Use a tablet press or manual tablet-making tool to compress the mixture into tablets. Ensure that each tablet is uniformly sized and well-compressed to avoid crumbling.

- If a tablet press is not available, you can use a mortar and pestle to blend and compress the ingredients manually, though this method may be less precise.

4. **Drying**:

- Allow the tablets to air dry completely before storing them. Proper drying is essential to prevent moisture from causing the tablets to break down. Place them on a clean, dry surface and let them dry for several hours or according to the tablet press instructions.

5. **Storage**:

- Store the dried tablets in airtight containers to protect them from moisture, light, and air. Keep the containers in a cool, dry place to maintain the tablets' potency and shelf life.

- Label the containers with the preparation date and any relevant information.

Dosage and Usage

- **Recommended Dosage**: Typically, 1-2 tablets per day are sufficient for supporting digestive health, but dosage may vary based on the tablets' potency and individual needs. Consult with a healthcare provider for personalized dosage recommendations.

- **Usage Instructions**: Take the tablets with a glass of water, preferably between meals. Regular use can help alleviate digestive discomfort, reduce bloating, and support overall gastrointestinal health.

Quality Control

- **Check for Uniformity**: Ensure that the tablets are of consistent size and weight for accurate dosing. Inspect the tablets for any signs of physical damage or degradation.

- **Potency Testing**: Periodically test the potency of the tablets to confirm they contain the intended levels of active ingredients.

Conclusion

Marshmallow root and caraway tablets offer a natural and effective way to support digestive health and soothe the gastrointestinal tract. By following the preparation and storage guidelines, you can create high-quality herbal tablets that harness the therapeutic benefits of these herbs, promoting overall well-being and digestive comfort.

Stress and Anxiety Relief

Chamomile and Lemon Balm Tablets

Chamomile and lemon balm are renowned for their calming and soothing properties, making them excellent choices for creating herbal tablets designed to alleviate stress, anxiety, and promote relaxation. This section provides a comprehensive guide to preparing effective chamomile and lemon balm tablets.

Benefits of Chamomile and Lemon Balm

- **Chamomile**: Chamomile is well-known for its gentle sedative effects, which help to reduce anxiety, promote relaxation, and improve sleep quality. It is particularly effective in calming the nervous system and can be beneficial for easing mild to moderate stress and promoting overall well-being.

- **Lemon Balm**: Lemon balm is celebrated for its calming and mood-enhancing effects. It helps to reduce symptoms of anxiety, support emotional balance, and improve cognitive function. Lemon balm also has mild sedative properties that can assist in promoting restful sleep and reducing nervous tension.

Ingredients

- **Chamomile Flower Powder**: Promotes relaxation, reduces anxiety, and improves sleep quality.

- **Lemon Balm Leaf Powder**: Reduces anxiety, supports emotional balance, and enhances cognitive function.

- **Binder**: Such as cellulose powder or starch, to ensure proper tablet formation.

- **Optional Additives**: Natural flavorings or sweeteners, if desired, to enhance taste.

Preparation Process

1. **Gather Ingredients**:

   - **Chamomile Flower Powder**: 50%

   - **Lemon Balm Leaf Powder**: 40%

   - **Binder**: 10% (such as cellulose powder or starch)

2. **Mixing**:

- In a clean, dry bowl, combine the chamomile flower powder and lemon balm leaf powder. Stir thoroughly to ensure an even distribution of both powders.

- Gradually add the binder to the mixture. The binder helps the herbs adhere together and ensures that the tablets hold their shape and consistency.

3. **Forming Tablets**:

- Use a tablet press or manual tablet-making tool to compress the mixture into tablets. Ensure that each tablet is uniformly sized and well-compressed to avoid crumbling.

- If a tablet press is not available, you can use a mortar and pestle to blend and compress the ingredients manually, though this method may be less precise.

4. **Drying**:

- Allow the tablets to air dry completely before storing them. Proper drying is essential to prevent moisture from causing the tablets to break down. Place them on a clean, dry surface and let

them dry for several hours or according to the tablet press instructions.

5. **Storage**:

   o Store the dried tablets in airtight containers to protect them from moisture, light, and air. Keep the containers in a cool, dry place to maintain the tablets' potency and shelf life.

   o Label the containers with the preparation date and any relevant information.

Dosage and Usage

- **Recommended Dosage**: Typically, 1-2 tablets per day are sufficient for managing stress and promoting relaxation, but dosage may vary based on the tablets' potency and individual needs. Consult with a healthcare provider for personalized dosage recommendations.

- **Usage Instructions**: Take the tablets with a glass of water, preferably in the evening or before bedtime. Regular use can help reduce symptoms of anxiety, promote relaxation, and improve sleep quality.

Quality Control

- **Check for Uniformity**: Ensure that the tablets are of consistent size and weight for accurate dosing. Inspect the tablets for any signs of physical damage or degradation.

- **Potency Testing**: Periodically test the potency of the tablets to confirm they contain the intended levels of active ingredients.

Conclusion

Chamomile and lemon balm tablets offer a natural and effective solution for managing stress, anxiety, and promoting relaxation. By following the preparation and storage guidelines, you can create high-quality herbal tablets that harness the calming and therapeutic benefits of these herbs, helping to enhance overall mental well-being and improve sleep quality.

Ashwagandha and Valerian Root Tablets

Ashwagandha and valerian root are two powerful herbs known for their stress-relieving and calming properties. Combining these herbs into tablet form can create an effective remedy for managing stress, anxiety, and promoting relaxation. This section provides a comprehensive guide to preparing high-quality ashwagandha and valerian root tablets.

Benefits of Ashwagandha and Valerian Root

- **Ashwagandha**: Ashwagandha is an adaptogenic herb that helps the body adapt to stress and restore balance. It supports adrenal function, reduces cortisol levels, and promotes a sense of calm and resilience. Ashwagandha is also known for its mood-stabilizing effects, making it beneficial for reducing symptoms of anxiety and improving overall mental well-being.

- **Valerian Root**: Valerian root is well-regarded for its ability to induce relaxation and improve sleep quality. It has sedative properties that help calm the nervous system and alleviate symptoms of anxiety. Valerian root is effective for managing stress-related insomnia and supporting restful sleep.

Ingredients

- **Ashwagandha Root Powder**: Supports stress adaptation, reduces cortisol levels, and promotes calm.

- **Valerian Root Powder**: Provides relaxation, improves sleep quality, and alleviates anxiety.

- **Binder**: Such as cellulose powder or starch, to ensure proper tablet formation.

- **Optional Additives**: Natural flavorings or sweeteners, if desired, to enhance taste.

Preparation Process

1. **Gather Ingredients**:

   - **Ashwagandha Root Powder**: 50%

   - **Valerian Root Powder**: 40%

   - **Binder**: 10% (such as cellulose powder or starch)

2. **Mixing**:

   - In a clean, dry bowl, combine the ashwagandha root powder and valerian root powder. Stir thoroughly to ensure an even distribution of both powders.

   - Gradually add the binder to the mixture. The binder helps the herbs adhere together and ensures that the tablets maintain their shape and consistency.

3. **Forming Tablets**:

- Use a tablet press or manual tablet-making tool to compress the mixture into tablets. Ensure that each tablet is uniformly sized and well-compressed to avoid crumbling.

- If a tablet press is not available, you can use a mortar and pestle to blend and compress the ingredients manually, though this method may be less precise.

4. **Drying**:

- Allow the tablets to air dry completely before storing them. Proper drying prevents moisture from causing the tablets to degrade. Place them on a clean, dry surface and let them dry for several hours or according to the tablet press instructions.

5. **Storage**:

- Store the dried tablets in airtight containers to protect them from moisture, light, and air. Keep the containers in a cool, dry place to maintain the tablets' potency and shelf life.

- Label the containers with the preparation date and any relevant information.

Dosage and Usage

- **Recommended Dosage**: Typically, 1-2 tablets per day are sufficient for managing stress and promoting relaxation, but dosage may vary based on the tablets' potency and individual needs. Consult with a healthcare provider for personalized dosage recommendations.

- **Usage Instructions**: Take the tablets with a glass of water, preferably in the evening or before bedtime. Regular use can help reduce symptoms of anxiety, promote relaxation, and improve sleep quality.

Quality Control

- **Check for Uniformity**: Ensure that the tablets are of consistent size and weight for accurate dosing. Inspect the tablets for any signs of physical damage or degradation.

- **Potency Testing**: Periodically test the potency of the tablets to confirm they contain the intended levels of active ingredients.

Conclusion

Ashwagandha and valerian root tablets provide a natural and effective approach to managing stress and anxiety while promoting relaxation and restful sleep. By following the preparation and storage guidelines, you can create high-quality herbal tablets that utilize the therapeutic benefits of these herbs, helping to enhance overall mental well-being and support a more balanced and relaxed state.

Passionflower and Kava Kava Tablets

Passionflower and kava kava are both renowned for their calming and anxiety-reducing properties. Combining these herbs into tablet form creates an effective remedy for managing stress and promoting relaxation. This section provides a comprehensive guide to preparing high-quality passionflower and kava kava tablets.

Benefits of Passionflower and Kava Kava

- **Passionflower**: Passionflower is known for its ability to soothe the nervous system and alleviate symptoms of anxiety and insomnia. It promotes relaxation and supports a restful night's sleep. Passionflower's gentle sedative effects help calm the mind and reduce feelings of tension and restlessness.

- **Kava Kava**: Kava kava is recognized for its powerful anxiolytic effects, making it effective for reducing anxiety and promoting relaxation. It helps relax the mind and body without impairing cognitive function, making it a valuable herb for managing stress and enhancing overall mood. Kava kava is also used to promote a sense of well-being and calmness.

Ingredients

- **Passionflower Powder**: Reduces anxiety, promotes relaxation, and improves sleep quality.

- **Kava Kava Root Powder**: Alleviates anxiety, supports relaxation, and enhances mood.

- **Binder**: Such as cellulose powder or starch, to ensure proper tablet formation.

- **Optional Additives**: Natural flavorings or sweeteners, if desired, to enhance taste.

Preparation Process

1. **Gather Ingredients**:

   - **Passionflower Powder**: 50%

   - **Kava Kava Root Powder**: 40%

   - **Binder**: 10% (such as cellulose powder or starch)

2. **Mixing**:

- In a clean, dry bowl, combine the passionflower powder and kava kava root powder. Stir thoroughly to ensure an even distribution of both powders.

- Gradually add the binder to the mixture. The binder helps the herbs adhere together and ensures that the tablets maintain their shape and consistency.

3. **Forming Tablets**:

- Use a tablet press or manual tablet-making tool to compress the mixture into tablets. Ensure that each tablet is uniformly sized and well-compressed to avoid crumbling.

- If a tablet press is not available, you can use a mortar and pestle to blend and compress the ingredients manually, though this method may be less precise.

4. **Drying**:

- Allow the tablets to air dry completely before storing them. Proper drying is essential to prevent moisture from causing the tablets to break down. Place them on a clean, dry surface and let

them dry for several hours or according to the tablet press instructions.

5. **Storage**:

   ○ Store the dried tablets in airtight containers to protect them from moisture, light, and air. Keep the containers in a cool, dry place to maintain the tablets' potency and shelf life.

   ○ Label the containers with the preparation date and any relevant information.

Dosage and Usage

- **Recommended Dosage**: Typically, 1-2 tablets per day are sufficient for managing stress and promoting relaxation, but dosage may vary based on the tablets' potency and individual needs. Consult with a healthcare provider for personalized dosage recommendations.

- **Usage Instructions**: Take the tablets with a glass of water, preferably in the evening or before bedtime. Regular use can help reduce symptoms of anxiety, support relaxation, and enhance overall mood.

Quality Control

- **Check for Uniformity**: Ensure that the tablets are of consistent size and weight for accurate dosing. Inspect the tablets for any signs of physical damage or degradation.

- **Potency Testing**: Periodically test the potency of the tablets to confirm they contain the intended levels of active ingredients.

Conclusion

Passionflower and kava kava tablets offer a natural and effective approach to managing stress and anxiety while promoting relaxation and enhancing mood. By following the preparation and storage guidelines, you can create high-quality herbal tablets that leverage the calming and therapeutic benefits of these herbs, helping to improve overall well-being and support a more balanced state of mind.

Rhodiola and Holy Basil Tablets

Rhodiola and holy basil are potent herbs known for their adaptogenic and stress-relieving properties. Combining these herbs into tablet form creates a powerful remedy for enhancing resilience to stress, improving mental clarity, and promoting overall well-being. This section provides a comprehensive guide to preparing effective rhodiola and holy basil tablets.

Benefits of Rhodiola and Holy Basil

- **Rhodiola**: Rhodiola is an adaptogen that helps the body adapt to stress and enhances mental and physical endurance. It improves mood, reduces fatigue, and supports cognitive function. Rhodiola is particularly useful for combating the effects of chronic stress and boosting overall vitality.

- **Holy Basil**: Holy basil, also known as tulsi, is another adaptogenic herb that helps manage stress and support mental clarity. It balances cortisol levels, reduces anxiety, and promotes a sense of calm. Holy basil also has anti-inflammatory and immune-boosting properties, making it beneficial for overall health and resilience.

Ingredients

- **Rhodiola Root Powder**: Enhances resilience to stress, reduces fatigue, and supports cognitive function.

- **Holy Basil Leaf Powder**: Balances stress hormones, reduces anxiety, and promotes mental clarity.

- **Binder**: Such as cellulose powder or starch, to ensure proper tablet formation.

- **Optional Additives**: Natural flavorings or sweeteners, if desired, to enhance taste.

Preparation Process

1. **Gather Ingredients**:

   - **Rhodiola Root Powder**: 50%

   - **Holy Basil Leaf Powder**: 40%

   - **Binder**: 10% (such as cellulose powder or starch)

2. **Mixing**:

   - In a clean, dry bowl, combine the rhodiola root powder and holy basil leaf powder. Stir thoroughly to ensure an even distribution of both powders.

   - Gradually add the binder to the mixture. The binder helps the herbs adhere together and ensures that the tablets maintain their shape and consistency.

3. **Forming Tablets**:

- Use a tablet press or manual tablet-making tool to compress the mixture into tablets. Ensure that each tablet is uniformly sized and well-compressed to avoid crumbling.

- If a tablet press is not available, you can use a mortar and pestle to blend and compress the ingredients manually, though this method may be less precise.

4. **Drying**:

- Allow the tablets to air dry completely before storing them. Proper drying is essential to prevent moisture from causing the tablets to break down. Place them on a clean, dry surface and let them dry for several hours or according to the tablet press instructions.

5. **Storage**:

- Store the dried tablets in airtight containers to protect them from moisture, light, and air. Keep the containers in a cool, dry place to maintain the tablets' potency and shelf life.

- Label the containers with the preparation date and any relevant information.

Dosage and Usage

- **Recommended Dosage**: Typically, 1-2 tablets per day are sufficient for enhancing resilience to stress and improving mental clarity, but dosage may vary based on the tablets' potency and individual needs. Consult with a healthcare provider for personalized dosage recommendations.

- **Usage Instructions**: Take the tablets with a glass of water, preferably in the morning or early afternoon. Regular use can help manage stress, boost energy levels, and support overall mental and physical health.

Quality Control

- **Check for Uniformity**: Ensure that the tablets are of consistent size and weight for accurate dosing. Inspect the tablets for any signs of physical damage or degradation.

- **Potency Testing**: Periodically test the potency of the tablets to confirm they contain the intended levels of active ingredients.

Conclusion

Rhodiola and holy basil tablets offer a natural and effective way to enhance stress resilience, improve mental clarity, and support overall well-being. By following the preparation and storage guidelines, you can create high-quality herbal tablets that utilize the adaptogenic benefits of these herbs, helping to promote a balanced and healthy state of mind and body.

Pain and Inflammation Management

Turmeric and Boswellia Tablets

Turmeric and boswellia are two powerful herbs renowned for their anti-inflammatory and pain-relieving properties. Combining these herbs into tablet form provides a natural remedy for managing inflammation and discomfort associated with various conditions. This section outlines how to create effective turmeric and boswellia tablets for pain and inflammation management.

Benefits of Turmeric and Boswellia

- **Turmeric**: Turmeric contains curcumin, a compound with strong anti-inflammatory and antioxidant properties. It helps reduce inflammation and alleviate pain, particularly useful for conditions such as arthritis, joint pain, and muscle soreness. Turmeric also supports overall joint health and mobility.

- **Boswellia**: Boswellia, or frankincense, is known for its potent anti-inflammatory effects. It supports joint health, reduces pain, and alleviates symptoms associated with inflammatory conditions like osteoarthritis and rheumatoid arthritis. Boswellia also helps improve flexibility and overall joint function.

Ingredients

- **Turmeric Root Powder**: Contains curcumin, which helps reduce inflammation and pain.

- **Boswellia Resin Powder**: Provides anti-inflammatory benefits and supports joint health.

- **Binder**: Such as cellulose powder or starch, to ensure proper tablet formation.

- **Optional Additives**: Natural flavorings or sweeteners, if desired, to enhance taste.

Preparation Process

1. **Gather Ingredients**:

   o **Turmeric Root Powder**: 50%

   o **Boswellia Resin Powder**: 40%

   o **Binder**: 10% (such as cellulose powder or starch)

2. **Mixing**:

   o In a clean, dry bowl, combine the turmeric root powder and boswellia resin powder. Stir thoroughly to ensure an even distribution of both powders.

   o Gradually add the binder to the mixture. The binder helps the herbs adhere together and ensures that the tablets maintain their shape and consistency.

3. **Forming Tablets**:

   o Use a tablet press or manual tablet-making tool to compress the mixture into tablets. Ensure that each tablet is uniformly sized and well-compressed to avoid crumbling.

   o If a tablet press is not available, you can use a mortar and pestle to blend and compress the ingredients manually, though this method may be less precise.

4. **Drying**:

   o Allow the tablets to air dry completely before storing them. Proper drying is essential to prevent moisture from causing the tablets to break down. Place them on a clean, dry surface and let

them dry for several hours or according to the tablet press instructions.

5. **Storage**:

   - Store the dried tablets in airtight containers to protect them from moisture, light, and air. Keep the containers in a cool, dry place to maintain the tablets' potency and shelf life.

   - Label the containers with the preparation date and any relevant information.

Dosage and Usage

- **Recommended Dosage**: Typically, 1-2 tablets per day are sufficient for managing inflammation and pain, but dosage may vary based on the tablets' potency and individual needs. Consult with a healthcare provider for personalized dosage recommendations.

- **Usage Instructions**: Take the tablets with a glass of water, preferably with meals or as needed for pain relief. Regular use can help manage symptoms of inflammation and discomfort, supporting overall joint health and mobility.

Quality Control

- **Check for Uniformity**: Ensure that the tablets are of consistent size and weight for accurate dosing. Inspect the tablets for any signs of physical damage or degradation.

- **Potency Testing**: Periodically test the potency of the tablets to confirm they contain the intended levels of active ingredients.

Conclusion

Turmeric and boswellia tablets offer a natural and effective approach to managing inflammation and pain. By harnessing the anti-inflammatory and pain-relieving properties of turmeric and boswellia, you can create high-quality herbal tablets that support joint health, reduce discomfort, and enhance overall well-being. Following the preparation and storage guidelines will help maintain the potency and effectiveness of your tablets, providing a valuable tool for managing inflammation and promoting comfort.

Willow Bark and Arnica Tablets

Willow bark and arnica are well-regarded for their natural pain-relieving and anti-inflammatory properties. Combining these herbs into tablet form provides an effective remedy for managing pain, reducing inflammation, and supporting overall musculoskeletal health. This section offers a comprehensive guide to creating willow bark and arnica tablets.

Benefits of Willow Bark and Arnica

- **Willow Bark**: Willow bark contains salicin, a compound with properties similar to aspirin. It is known for its effectiveness in alleviating pain and reducing inflammation. Willow bark is particularly beneficial for conditions such as joint pain, back pain, and headaches.

- **Arnica**: Arnica is commonly used for its anti-inflammatory and pain-relieving effects. It helps reduce bruising, swelling, and muscle soreness. Arnica is especially useful for treating localized pain, such as that resulting from minor injuries or strains.

Ingredients

- **Willow Bark Powder**: Provides natural pain relief and anti-inflammatory benefits.

- **Arnica Flower Powder**: Reduces inflammation, relieves pain, and supports recovery from minor injuries.

- **Binder**: Such as cellulose powder or starch, to ensure proper tablet formation.

- **Optional Additives**: Natural flavorings or sweeteners, if desired, to enhance taste.

Preparation Process

1. **Gather Ingredients**:

   - **Willow Bark Powder**: 50%

   - **Arnica Flower Powder**: 40%

   - **Binder**: 10% (such as cellulose powder or starch)

2. **Mixing**:

   - In a clean, dry bowl, combine the willow bark powder and arnica flower powder. Stir thoroughly to ensure an even distribution of both powders.

   - Gradually add the binder to the mixture. The binder helps the herbs adhere together and ensures that the tablets maintain their shape and consistency.

3. **Forming Tablets**:

- Use a tablet press or manual tablet-making tool to compress the mixture into tablets. Ensure that each tablet is uniformly sized and well-compressed to avoid crumbling.

- If a tablet press is not available, you can use a mortar and pestle to blend and compress the ingredients manually, though this method may be less precise.

4. **Drying**:

- Allow the tablets to air dry completely before storing them. Proper drying is essential to prevent moisture from causing the tablets to break down. Place them on a clean, dry surface and let them dry for several hours or according to the tablet press instructions.

5. **Storage**:

- Store the dried tablets in airtight containers to protect them from moisture, light, and air. Keep the containers in a cool, dry place to maintain the tablets' potency and shelf life.

- Label the containers with the preparation date and any relevant information.

Dosage and Usage

- **Recommended Dosage**: Typically, 1-2 tablets per day are sufficient for managing pain and inflammation, but dosage may vary based on the tablets' potency and individual needs. Consult with a healthcare provider for personalized dosage recommendations.

- **Usage Instructions**: Take the tablets with a glass of water, preferably with meals or as needed for pain relief. Regular use can help manage symptoms of pain and inflammation, supporting overall comfort and recovery.

Quality Control

- **Check for Uniformity**: Ensure that the tablets are of consistent size and weight for accurate dosing. Inspect the tablets for any signs of physical damage or degradation.

- **Potency Testing**: Periodically test the potency of the tablets to confirm they contain the intended levels of active ingredients.

Conclusion

Willow bark and arnica tablets provide a natural approach to managing pain and inflammation. By leveraging the analgesic and anti-inflammatory properties of willow bark and arnica, you can create effective herbal tablets that support pain relief, reduce inflammation, and promote recovery from minor injuries. Following the preparation and storage guidelines will help maintain the potency and effectiveness of your tablets, offering a valuable tool for managing discomfort and enhancing overall well-being.

Ginger and Devil's Claw Tablets

Ginger and devil's claw are powerful herbs known for their anti-inflammatory and pain-relieving properties. Combining these herbs into tablet form creates a natural remedy effective in managing pain, reducing inflammation, and supporting joint and digestive health. This section provides a comprehensive guide to preparing ginger and devil's claw tablets.

Benefits of Ginger and Devil's Claw

- **Ginger**: Ginger contains active compounds such as gingerol and shogaol, which possess strong anti-inflammatory and analgesic properties. It is widely used to alleviate digestive issues, reduce nausea, and relieve muscle and joint pain. Ginger also helps in managing symptoms of osteoarthritis and rheumatoid arthritis.

- **Devil's Claw**: Devil's claw, derived from the root of Harpagophytum procumbens, is renowned for its potent anti-inflammatory and pain-relieving effects. It is particularly beneficial for managing joint pain, arthritis, and lower back pain. Devil's claw supports joint health and reduces symptoms associated with chronic inflammatory conditions.

Ingredients

- **Ginger Root Powder**: Provides anti-inflammatory and analgesic benefits, helps relieve digestive issues and muscle pain.

- **Devil's Claw Root Powder**: Reduces inflammation and alleviates joint and back pain.

- **Binder**: Such as cellulose powder or starch, to ensure proper tablet formation.

- **Optional Additives**: Natural flavorings or sweeteners, if desired, to enhance taste.

Preparation Process

1. **Gather Ingredients**:

   - **Ginger Root Powder**: 50%

   - **Devil's Claw Root Powder**: 40%

- **Binder**: 10% (such as cellulose powder or starch)

2. **Mixing**:

   - In a clean, dry bowl, combine the ginger root powder and devil's claw root powder. Stir thoroughly to ensure an even distribution of both powders.

   - Gradually add the binder to the mixture. The binder helps the powders adhere together and ensures that the tablets maintain their shape and consistency.

3. **Forming Tablets**:

   - Use a tablet press or manual tablet-making tool to compress the mixture into tablets. Ensure that each tablet is uniformly sized and well-compressed to avoid crumbling.

   - If a tablet press is not available, you can use a mortar and pestle to blend and compress the ingredients manually, though this method may be less precise.

4. **Drying**:

   - Allow the tablets to air dry completely before storing them. Proper drying is essential to prevent moisture from causing the tablets to break down. Place them on a clean, dry surface and let them dry for several hours or according to the tablet press instructions.

5. **Storage**:

   o Store the dried tablets in airtight containers to protect them from moisture, light, and air. Keep the containers in a cool, dry place to maintain the tablets' potency and shelf life.

   o Label the containers with the preparation date and any relevant information.

Dosage and Usage

- **Recommended Dosage**: Typically, 1-2 tablets per day are sufficient for managing pain and inflammation, but dosage may vary based on the tablets' potency and individual needs. Consult with a healthcare provider for personalized dosage recommendations.

- **Usage Instructions**: Take the tablets with a glass of water, preferably with meals or as needed for pain relief and digestive support. Regular use can help manage symptoms of inflammation and discomfort, supporting overall health and well-being.

Quality Control

- **Check for Uniformity**: Ensure that the tablets are of consistent size and weight for accurate dosing. Inspect the tablets for any signs of physical damage or degradation.

- **Potency Testing**: Periodically test the potency of the tablets to confirm they contain the intended levels of active ingredients.

Conclusion

Ginger and devil's claw tablets offer a natural solution for managing pain and inflammation while supporting digestive health. By utilizing the anti-inflammatory and analgesic properties of ginger and devil's claw, you can create effective herbal tablets that help alleviate discomfort, support joint health, and promote overall well-being. Following the preparation and storage guidelines will help maintain the potency and effectiveness of your tablets, providing a valuable tool for natural pain management and health support.

Capsaicin and Pineapple Enzyme Tablets

Capsaicin and pineapple enzyme (bromelain) are two herbs known for their unique properties that can aid in pain relief and inflammation reduction. Combining these herbs into tablet form provides a powerful natural remedy for managing pain, supporting digestive health, and promoting overall well-being. This section offers a comprehensive guide to preparing capsaicin and pineapple enzyme tablets.

Benefits of Capsaicin and Pineapple Enzyme

- **Capsaicin**: Capsaicin is the active compound found in chili peppers that gives them their heat. It has well-documented analgesic properties, making it effective in managing pain associated with arthritis, muscle strains, and neuropathy. Capsaicin works by desensitizing pain receptors, which helps reduce the sensation of pain over time.

- **Pineapple Enzyme (Bromelain)**: Bromelain is an enzyme derived from pineapple stems and fruit. It has anti-inflammatory properties and supports digestion by breaking down proteins. Bromelain can help reduce swelling, bruising, and pain related to inflammation. It is particularly useful for managing symptoms of arthritis and promoting digestive health.

Ingredients

- **Capsaicin Powder**: Provides pain relief by desensitizing pain receptors and reducing inflammation.

- **Pineapple Enzyme Powder (Bromelain)**: Supports anti-inflammatory responses and aids digestion.

- **Binder**: Such as cellulose powder or starch, to ensure proper tablet formation.

- **Optional Additives**: Natural flavorings or sweeteners, if desired, to enhance taste.

Preparation Process

1. **Gather Ingredients**:

   - **Capsaicin Powder**: 30%

   - **Pineapple Enzyme Powder (Bromelain)**: 50%

   - **Binder**: 20% (such as cellulose powder or starch)

2. **Mixing**:

   - In a clean, dry bowl, combine the capsaicin powder and pineapple enzyme powder. Stir thoroughly to ensure an even distribution of both powders.

o   Gradually add the binder to the mixture. The binder helps the powders adhere together and ensures that the tablets maintain their shape and consistency.

3. **Forming Tablets**:

   o   Use a tablet press or manual tablet-making tool to compress the mixture into tablets. Ensure that each tablet is uniformly sized and well-compressed to avoid crumbling.

   o   If a tablet press is not available, you can use a mortar and pestle to blend and compress the ingredients manually, though this method may be less precise.

4. **Drying**:

   o   Allow the tablets to air dry completely before storing them. Proper drying is essential to prevent moisture from causing the tablets to break down. Place them on a clean, dry surface and let them dry for several hours or according to the tablet press instructions.

5. **Storage**:

- Store the dried tablets in airtight containers to protect them from moisture, light, and air. Keep the containers in a cool, dry place to maintain the tablets' potency and shelf life.

- Label the containers with the preparation date and any relevant information.

Dosage and Usage

- **Recommended Dosage**: Typically, 1-2 tablets per day are sufficient for managing pain and supporting digestive health, but dosage may vary based on the tablets' potency and individual needs. Consult with a healthcare provider for personalized dosage recommendations.

- **Usage Instructions**: Take the tablets with a glass of water, preferably with meals or as needed for pain relief and digestive support. Regular use can help manage symptoms of inflammation, pain, and digestive discomfort.

Quality Control

- **Check for Uniformity**: Ensure that the tablets are of consistent size and weight for accurate dosing. Inspect the tablets for any signs of physical damage or degradation.

- **Potency Testing**: Periodically test the potency of the tablets to confirm they contain the intended levels of active ingredients.

Conclusion

Capsaicin and pineapple enzyme tablets offer a natural approach to managing pain, reducing inflammation, and supporting digestive health. By harnessing the therapeutic properties of capsaicin and bromelain, you can create effective herbal tablets that provide relief from discomfort and support overall wellness. Following the preparation and storage guidelines will help maintain the potency and effectiveness of your tablets, offering a valuable tool for natural health management.

Chapter 5: Specialized Herbal Tablets

For Respiratory Health

Mullein and Thyme Tablets

Mullein and thyme are two herbs renowned for their benefits to respiratory health. Combining these herbs into tablet form offers a natural remedy for respiratory issues such as coughs, congestion, and inflammation. This section provides a detailed guide on preparing mullein and thyme tablets.

Benefits of Mullein and Thyme

- **Mullein**: Mullein is traditionally used to soothe and heal the respiratory tract. It has anti-inflammatory properties that can reduce irritation and inflammation in the lungs and throat. Mullein helps ease coughs and bronchial congestion by acting as an expectorant, promoting the expulsion of mucus.

- **Thyme**: Thyme is known for its antimicrobial and expectorant qualities. It can help clear mucus from the respiratory passages and soothe coughing. Thyme's antiseptic properties also support respiratory health by reducing bacterial and viral infections.

Ingredients

- **Mullein Leaf Powder**: Provides soothing and anti-inflammatory benefits for the respiratory system.

- **Thyme Leaf Powder**: Offers antimicrobial and expectorant properties to support respiratory health.

- **Binder**: Such as cellulose powder or starch to ensure proper tablet formation.

- **Optional Additives**: Natural flavorings or sweeteners, if desired, to improve taste.

Preparation Process

1. **Gather Ingredients**:

   - **Mullein Leaf Powder**: 50%

   - **Thyme Leaf Powder**: 40%

   - **Binder**: 10% (e.g., cellulose powder or starch)

2. **Mixing**:

- In a clean, dry bowl, combine the mullein leaf powder and thyme leaf powder. Stir thoroughly to ensure even distribution of the herbs.

- Gradually add the binder to the mixture and mix well until the binder is fully integrated.

3. **Forming Tablets:**

- Use a tablet press or manual tablet-making tool to compress the mixture into tablets. Ensure that each tablet is uniform in size and well-compressed to maintain integrity and consistency.

4. **Drying:**

- Allow the tablets to air dry completely before storing. Place them on a clean, dry surface to prevent any moisture from affecting the tablets.

5. **Storage:**

- Store the dried tablets in airtight containers to protect them from moisture, light, and air. Keep the containers in a cool, dry place to maintain the tablets' potency and shelf life.

- Label the containers with the preparation date and the contents of the tablets.

Dosage and Usage

- **Recommended Dosage**: Generally, 1-2 tablets per day are recommended, but the dosage may vary based on individual needs and the potency of the tablets. Consult a healthcare provider for personalized dosage instructions.

- **Usage Instructions**: Take the tablets with a glass of water. They can be taken with meals or as needed to support respiratory health and alleviate symptoms of coughs and congestion.

Quality Control

- **Check for Uniformity**: Ensure that the tablets are consistently sized and weighted to provide accurate dosing.

- **Potency Testing**: Periodically test the tablets to confirm that they contain the intended levels of active ingredients. This ensures that the tablets are effective and safe for use.

Conclusion

Mullein and thyme tablets offer a natural solution for supporting respiratory health and managing symptoms related to coughs, congestion, and inflammation. By combining the soothing and antimicrobial properties of these herbs, you can create an effective herbal remedy that promotes respiratory wellness. Following the preparation and storage guidelines will help ensure that your tablets maintain their potency and effectiveness, providing valuable support for respiratory health.

Licorice Root and Marshmallow Tablets

Licorice root and marshmallow root are renowned for their soothing properties and ability to support respiratory and digestive health. Combining these herbs into tablet form provides a natural remedy for conditions such as throat irritation, coughs, and digestive discomfort. Here's a detailed guide on preparing licorice root and marshmallow tablets.

Benefits of Licorice Root and Marshmallow Root

- **Licorice Root**: Known for its anti-inflammatory and soothing properties, licorice root helps alleviate throat irritation and coughs. It also supports digestive health by reducing inflammation and promoting mucous membrane health in the digestive tract.

- **Marshmallow Root**: Marshmallow root is traditionally used to soothe mucous membranes and reduce inflammation. It is especially beneficial for calming irritated tissues in the throat and digestive tract, making it an excellent complement to licorice root in addressing respiratory and digestive discomfort.

Ingredients

- **Licorice Root Powder**: Provides anti-inflammatory and soothing benefits for the throat and digestive system.

- **Marshmallow Root Powder**: Offers mucous membrane soothing and anti-inflammatory properties.

- **Binder**: Such as cellulose powder or starch to ensure proper tablet formation.

- **Optional Additives**: Natural flavorings or sweeteners, if desired, to enhance taste.

Preparation Process

1. **Gather Ingredients**:

   - **Licorice Root Powder**: 50%

   - **Marshmallow Root Powder**: 40%

- **Binder**: 10% (e.g., cellulose powder or starch)

2. **Mixing**:

   - In a clean, dry bowl, combine the licorice root powder and marshmallow root powder. Stir thoroughly to ensure an even blend of the herbs.

   - Gradually add the binder to the mixture and mix well until the binder is fully incorporated. This ensures that the herbs will be held together properly when compressed into tablets.

3. **Forming Tablets**:

   - Use a tablet press or manual tablet-making tool to compress the herb mixture into tablets. Ensure that each tablet is uniform in size and adequately compressed to maintain its shape and effectiveness.

4. **Drying**:

   - Allow the tablets to air dry completely before storing them. Place them on a clean, dry surface to avoid moisture accumulation and ensure proper drying.

5. **Storage**:

- Store the dried tablets in airtight containers to protect them from moisture, light, and air. Keep the containers in a cool, dry place to preserve the tablets' potency and extend their shelf life.

- Label the containers with the preparation date and the contents to ensure easy identification.

Dosage and Usage

- **Recommended Dosage**: Typically, 1-2 tablets per day are suggested. However, the dosage may vary based on individual health needs and the strength of the tablets. Consult a healthcare provider for personalized dosage recommendations.

- **Usage Instructions**: Take the tablets with a glass of water. They can be consumed with meals or as needed to support throat and digestive health.

Quality Control

- **Check for Uniformity**: Verify that the tablets are consistently sized and weighted to ensure accurate dosing and effectiveness.

- **Potency Testing**: Regularly test the tablets to confirm that they contain the correct levels of active ingredients, ensuring that the tablets are both effective and safe for use.

Conclusion

Licorice root and marshmallow root tablets provide a natural and soothing remedy for managing throat irritation, coughs, and digestive discomfort. By combining the mucous membrane-soothing properties of marshmallow root with the anti-inflammatory benefits of licorice root, these tablets offer comprehensive support for respiratory and digestive health. Following the preparation and storage guidelines will help ensure that the tablets maintain their efficacy and quality, offering a valuable natural remedy for various health concerns.

Eucalyptus and Sage Tablets

Eucalyptus and sage are two powerful herbs with significant benefits for respiratory health. Eucalyptus helps clear mucus and ease breathing, while sage provides antimicrobial and anti-inflammatory support. Combining these herbs into tablets creates a natural remedy for respiratory discomfort and overall lung health.

Benefits of Eucalyptus and Sage

- **Eucalyptus**: Eucalyptus is well-known for its ability to clear congestion and promote easier breathing. Its active compounds, such as cineole, have expectorant properties that help loosen mucus and reduce coughing. Eucalyptus also has antimicrobial qualities that can support respiratory health.

- **Sage**: Sage is traditionally used for its antimicrobial, anti-inflammatory, and soothing properties. It can help reduce throat irritation, alleviate coughing, and support overall respiratory function. Sage's antioxidants also contribute to its health benefits.

Ingredients

- **Eucalyptus Leaf Powder**: Provides decongestant and expectorant benefits to support respiratory health.

- **Sage Leaf Powder**: Offers antimicrobial and anti-inflammatory properties to soothe the throat and reduce coughing.

- **Binder**: Such as cellulose powder or starch to ensure proper tablet formation.

- **Optional Additives**: Natural flavorings or sweeteners, if desired, to enhance the taste.

Preparation Process

1. **Gather Ingredients**:

   - **Eucalyptus Leaf Powder**: 50%

   - **Sage Leaf Powder**: 40%

   - **Binder**: 10% (e.g., cellulose powder or starch)

2. **Mixing**:

   - In a clean, dry bowl, blend the eucalyptus leaf powder and sage leaf powder. Stir thoroughly to ensure an even distribution of both herbs.

   - Gradually add the binder to the mixture, mixing well until the binder is fully incorporated.

3. **Forming Tablets**:

   - Use a tablet press or manual tablet-making tool to compress the herb mixture into tablets. Ensure uniform size and proper compression to maintain the tablets' integrity.

4. **Drying**:

   ○ Allow the tablets to air dry completely before storing. Place them on a clean, dry surface to ensure they dry thoroughly without moisture affecting them.

5. **Storage**:

   ○ Store the dried tablets in airtight containers to protect them from moisture, light, and air. Keep the containers in a cool, dry place to maintain the potency and shelf life of the tablets.

   ○ Label the containers with the preparation date and contents for easy identification.

Dosage and Usage

- **Recommended Dosage**: Typically, 1-2 tablets per day are suggested. However, the dosage may vary based on individual needs and the strength of the tablets. Consult a healthcare provider for personalized dosage recommendations.

- **Usage Instructions**: Take the tablets with a glass of water. They can be taken with meals or as needed to support respiratory health and alleviate symptoms of coughs and congestion.

Quality Control

- **Check for Uniformity**: Ensure that the tablets are consistently sized and weighted to provide accurate dosing and effectiveness.

- **Potency Testing**: Periodically test the tablets to confirm that they contain the intended levels of active ingredients, ensuring the tablets remain effective and safe for use.

Conclusion

Eucalyptus and sage tablets offer a natural solution for respiratory health, helping to clear congestion, soothe irritation, and support overall lung function. By combining the decongestant properties of eucalyptus with the antimicrobial and anti-inflammatory benefits of sage, these tablets provide comprehensive support for respiratory well-being. Adhering to the preparation and storage guidelines will help ensure that the tablets maintain their potency and effectiveness, offering a valuable remedy for respiratory discomfort.

Oregano and Lobelia Tablets

Oregano and lobelia are two potent herbs with complementary benefits for respiratory health and overall wellness. Oregano is known for its antimicrobial and anti-inflammatory properties, while lobelia helps support respiratory function and ease breathing. Combining these herbs into tablet form provides a natural remedy for respiratory discomfort and immune support.

Benefits of Oregano and Lobelia

- **Oregano**: Oregano is celebrated for its strong antimicrobial and antioxidant properties. It helps combat infections, reduce inflammation, and support overall respiratory health. Its active compounds, such as carvacrol, contribute to its ability to alleviate respiratory symptoms and boost the immune system.

- **Lobelia**: Lobelia has been used traditionally to support respiratory health by acting as an expectorant and bronchodilator. It helps to clear mucus from the respiratory tract, making it easier to breathe and alleviating symptoms of coughs and congestion.

Ingredients

- **Oregano Leaf Powder**: Provides antimicrobial, anti-inflammatory, and antioxidant benefits to support respiratory and immune health.

- **Lobelia Herb Powder**: Offers expectorant and bronchodilator properties to aid in respiratory function and mucus clearance.

- **Binder**: Such as cellulose powder or starch to ensure proper tablet formation.

- **Optional Additives**: Natural flavorings or sweeteners, if desired, to improve taste.

Preparation Process

1. **Gather Ingredients**:

   - **Oregano Leaf Powder**: 50%

   - **Lobelia Herb Powder**: 40%

   - **Binder**: 10% (e.g., cellulose powder or starch)

2. **Mixing**:

   - In a clean, dry bowl, combine the oregano leaf powder and lobelia herb powder. Stir thoroughly to ensure an even distribution of the herbs.

o   Gradually add the binder to the mixture and mix well until the binder is fully incorporated. This step ensures that the tablets will hold together properly.

3. **Forming Tablets**:

    o   Use a tablet press or manual tablet-making tool to compress the herb mixture into tablets. Ensure that each tablet is uniform in size and adequately compressed to maintain its shape and effectiveness.

4. **Drying**:

    o   Allow the tablets to air dry completely before storing them. Place them on a clean, dry surface to prevent moisture accumulation and ensure proper drying.

5. **Storage**:

    o   Store the dried tablets in airtight containers to protect them from moisture, light, and air. Keep the containers in a cool, dry place to preserve the potency and extend the shelf life of the tablets.

    o   Label the containers with the preparation date and the contents for easy identification.

Dosage and Usage

- **Recommended Dosage**: Typically, 1-2 tablets per day are suggested. However, dosage may vary based on individual health needs and the strength of the tablets. Consult a healthcare provider for personalized dosage recommendations.

- **Usage Instructions**: Take the tablets with a glass of water. They can be taken with meals or as needed to support respiratory health and boost immune function.

Quality Control

- **Check for Uniformity**: Ensure that the tablets are consistently sized and weighted to provide accurate dosing and effectiveness.

- **Potency Testing**: Regularly test the tablets to confirm they contain the correct levels of active ingredients, ensuring the tablets remain effective and safe for use.

Conclusion

Oregano and lobelia tablets offer a natural remedy for enhancing respiratory health and immune support. By combining the antimicrobial and anti-inflammatory properties of oregano with the expectorant and bronchodilator benefits of lobelia, these tablets provide a comprehensive approach to managing respiratory discomfort and promoting overall well-being. Adhering to the preparation and storage guidelines will help ensure the tablets maintain their potency and effectiveness, offering a valuable natural solution for respiratory and immune health.

For Cardiovascular Health

Hawthorn Berry and Garlic Tablets

Hawthorn berry and garlic are two potent herbs known for their benefits to cardiovascular health. Hawthorn berry is celebrated for its ability to support heart function and circulation, while garlic is renowned for its cholesterol-lowering and blood pressure-regulating properties. Combining these herbs into tablets provides a convenient and effective way to support heart health.

Benefits of Hawthorn Berry and Garlic

- **Hawthorn Berry**: Hawthorn is commonly used to strengthen the heart muscle, improve circulation, and lower blood pressure. Its active compounds, including flavonoids and oligomeric proanthocyanidins (OPCs), contribute to its heart-supportive effects.

- **Garlic**: Garlic is known for its cardiovascular benefits, including lowering cholesterol levels, reducing blood pressure, and improving overall heart function. Its key active component, allicin, has been shown to have significant heart-health benefits.

Ingredients

- **Hawthorn Berry Powder**: Provides heart-strengthening and circulation-boosting benefits.

- **Garlic Powder**: Offers cholesterol-lowering and blood pressure-regulating effects.

- **Binder**: Such as cellulose powder or starch to ensure proper tablet formation.

- **Optional Additives**: Natural flavorings or sweeteners, if desired, to enhance taste.

Preparation Process

1. **Gather Ingredients**:

   - **Hawthorn Berry Powder**: 50%

   - **Garlic Powder**: 40%

o **Binder**: 10% (e.g., cellulose powder or starch)

2. **Mixing**:

   o In a clean, dry bowl, thoroughly combine the hawthorn berry powder and garlic powder. Mix well to ensure an even distribution of both herbs.

   o Gradually add the binder to the herb mixture and stir until fully incorporated. This helps the tablet mixture hold together properly.

3. **Forming Tablets**:

   o Use a tablet press or manual tablet-making tool to compress the herb mixture into tablets. Ensure that the tablets are uniform in size and adequately compressed to maintain their shape and effectiveness.

4. **Drying**:

   o Allow the tablets to air dry completely on a clean, dry surface. Proper drying prevents moisture from affecting the tablets and ensures they remain stable.

5. **Storage**:

- Store the dried tablets in airtight containers to protect them from moisture, light, and air. Keep the containers in a cool, dry place to maintain the tablets' potency and extend their shelf life.

- Label the containers with the preparation date and contents for easy identification.

Dosage and Usage

- **Recommended Dosage**: Generally, 1-2 tablets per day are recommended. Dosage may vary based on individual health needs and the strength of the tablets. Consult with a healthcare provider for personalized dosage instructions.

- **Usage Instructions**: Take the tablets with a glass of water. They can be consumed with meals or as needed to support cardiovascular health.

Quality Control

- **Check for Uniformity**: Verify that the tablets are consistently sized and weighted to ensure accurate dosing and effectiveness.

- **Potency Testing**: Regularly test the tablets to confirm that they contain the correct levels of active ingredients, ensuring that the tablets are both effective and safe for use.

Conclusion

Hawthorn berry and garlic tablets provide a natural and effective remedy for supporting cardiovascular health. By combining the heart-strengthening properties of hawthorn berry with the cholesterol-lowering and blood pressure-regulating benefits of garlic, these tablets offer comprehensive support for heart function and circulation. Adhering to the preparation and storage guidelines will help ensure that the tablets maintain their potency and effectiveness, providing a valuable addition to a heart-healthy regimen.

Hawthorn Berry and Ginger Tablets

Hawthorn berry and ginger are two powerful herbs known for their supportive roles in cardiovascular health and digestive wellness. Hawthorn berry is celebrated for its benefits to heart function and circulation, while ginger is renowned for its anti-inflammatory and digestive-supportive properties. Combining these herbs into tablets offers a natural remedy to promote heart health and aid digestion.

Benefits of Hawthorn Berry and Ginger

- **Hawthorn Berry**: Hawthorn is traditionally used to strengthen the heart muscle, improve circulation, and lower blood pressure. It contains flavonoids and oligomeric proanthocyanidins (OPCs) that support cardiovascular health by improving blood flow and reducing symptoms of heart-related conditions.

- **Ginger**: Ginger is well-known for its anti-inflammatory, antioxidant, and digestive benefits. It helps reduce nausea, improve digestion, and may support cardiovascular health by improving circulation and reducing inflammation.

Ingredients

- **Hawthorn Berry Powder**: Provides cardiovascular support by enhancing heart function and circulation.

- **Ginger Powder**: Offers anti-inflammatory and digestive benefits, and supports overall wellness.

- **Binder**: Such as cellulose powder or starch to ensure proper tablet formation.

- **Optional Additives**: Natural flavorings or sweeteners, if desired, to enhance taste.

Preparation Process

1. **Gather Ingredients**:

- Hawthorn Berry Powder: 50%

- Ginger Powder: 40%

- Binder: 10% (e.g., cellulose powder or starch)

2. **Mixing**:

   - In a clean, dry bowl, combine the hawthorn berry powder and ginger powder thoroughly. Ensure an even distribution of both powders.

   - Gradually add the binder to the herb mixture, mixing well until the binder is fully incorporated. This step helps the tablet mixture hold together effectively.

3. **Forming Tablets**:

   - Use a tablet press or manual tablet-making tool to compress the herb mixture into tablets. Ensure uniform size and proper compression to maintain the tablets' shape and effectiveness.

4. **Drying**:

   - Allow the tablets to air dry completely on a clean, dry surface. Proper drying prevents moisture from affecting the tablets and ensures their stability.

5. **Storage**:

  ○ Store the dried tablets in airtight containers to protect them from moisture, light, and air. Keep the containers in a cool, dry place to maintain the potency and extend the shelf life of the tablets.

  ○ Label the containers with the preparation date and contents for easy identification.

Dosage and Usage

- **Recommended Dosage**: Typically, 1-2 tablets per day. However, individual needs may vary based on health conditions and tablet potency. Consult a healthcare provider for personalized dosage recommendations.

- **Usage Instructions**: Take the tablets with a glass of water. They can be consumed with meals or as needed to support cardiovascular health and digestive wellness.

Quality Control

- **Check for Uniformity**: Ensure that the tablets are consistently sized and weighted for accurate dosing and effectiveness.

- **Potency Testing**: Regularly test the tablets to confirm they contain the correct levels of active ingredients, ensuring they remain effective and safe for use.

Conclusion

Hawthorn berry and ginger tablets offer a natural remedy that supports both cardiovascular health and digestive function. By combining the heart-strengthening benefits of hawthorn berry with the anti-inflammatory and digestive-supportive properties of ginger, these tablets provide a comprehensive approach to promoting overall wellness. Following the preparation and storage guidelines will help maintain the tablets' potency and effectiveness, making them a valuable addition to a health-supportive regimen.

Gingko Biloba and Motherwort Tablets

Ginkgo biloba and motherwort are two herbs known for their benefits to cognitive function and emotional well-being. Ginkgo biloba is famed for its ability to enhance cognitive function and circulation, while motherwort is valued for its calming effects and support for heart health. Combining these herbs into tablets offers a natural remedy that promotes mental clarity and emotional balance.

Benefits of Ginkgo Biloba and Motherwort

- **Ginkgo Biloba**: Ginkgo biloba is widely used to improve cognitive function, enhance memory, and support overall brain health. It works by increasing blood flow to the brain and providing antioxidant protection, which may help improve mental clarity and reduce symptoms of cognitive decline.

- **Motherwort**: Motherwort is traditionally used to support emotional well-being and cardiovascular health. It has calming properties that can help alleviate stress and anxiety, while also supporting heart function by improving circulation and reducing palpitations.

Ingredients

- **Ginkgo Biloba Powder**: Provides cognitive support and improves circulation.

- **Motherwort Powder**: Offers calming effects and supports cardiovascular health.

- **Binder**: Such as cellulose powder or starch to ensure proper tablet formation.

- **Optional Additives**: Natural flavorings or sweeteners, if desired, to enhance taste.

Preparation Process

1. **Gather Ingredients**:

   o **Ginkgo Biloba Powder**: 50%

   o **Motherwort Powder**: 40%

   o **Binder**: 10% (e.g., cellulose powder or starch)

2. **Mixing**:

   o In a clean, dry bowl, combine the ginkgo biloba powder and motherwort powder. Stir thoroughly to ensure even distribution of both powders.

   o Gradually add the binder to the herb mixture and mix until fully incorporated. This step ensures that the tablets will hold together properly.

3. **Forming Tablets**:

- Use a tablet press or manual tablet-making tool to compress the herb mixture into tablets. Ensure that the tablets are uniform in size and adequately compressed to maintain their shape and effectiveness.

4. **Drying**:

   - Allow the tablets to air dry completely on a clean, dry surface. Proper drying is essential to prevent moisture from affecting the tablets and to ensure their stability.

5. **Storage**:

   - Store the dried tablets in airtight containers to protect them from moisture, light, and air. Keep the containers in a cool, dry place to maintain the tablets' potency and extend their shelf life.

   - Label the containers with the preparation date and contents for easy identification.

Dosage and Usage

- **Recommended Dosage**: Generally, 1-2 tablets per day. However, dosage may vary based on individual health needs and tablet potency.

Consult a healthcare provider for personalized dosage recommendations.

- **Usage Instructions**: Take the tablets with a glass of water. They can be consumed with meals or as needed to support cognitive function and emotional balance.

Quality Control

- **Check for Uniformity**: Ensure that the tablets are consistently sized and weighted to provide accurate dosing and effectiveness.

- **Potency Testing**: Regularly test the tablets to confirm they contain the correct levels of active ingredients, ensuring the tablets are both effective and safe for use.

Conclusion

Ginkgo biloba and motherwort tablets offer a natural remedy to support cognitive function and emotional well-being. By combining the brain-boosting benefits of ginkgo biloba with the calming and heart-supportive effects of motherwort, these tablets provide a holistic approach to enhancing mental clarity and managing stress. Adhering to the preparation and storage guidelines will help ensure the tablets maintain their potency and effectiveness, making them a valuable addition to a balanced health regimen.

Red Clover and CoQ10 Tablets

Red clover and Coenzyme Q10 (CoQ10) are two beneficial supplements that can support various aspects of health. Red clover is known for its benefits to hormone balance and cardiovascular health, while CoQ10 plays a crucial role in cellular energy production and antioxidant protection. Combining these two into tablets provides a convenient way to support overall wellness, from heart health to energy levels.

Benefits of Red Clover and CoQ10

- **Red Clover**: Red clover is often used to support hormonal balance, particularly in women, and to promote cardiovascular health. It contains isoflavones, which are plant compounds with estrogen-like effects that can help alleviate symptoms of menopause and support heart health by improving blood circulation and reducing cholesterol levels.

- **CoQ10**: Coenzyme Q10 is an essential nutrient that supports energy production in cells and acts as a powerful antioxidant. It helps protect cells from oxidative damage, supports heart health, and may improve energy levels and reduce fatigue.

Ingredients

- **Red Clover Powder**: Provides hormone-balancing and cardiovascular benefits.

- **CoQ10 Powder**: Supports cellular energy production and offers antioxidant protection.

- **Binder**: Such as cellulose powder or starch to ensure proper tablet formation.

- **Optional Additives**: Natural flavorings or sweeteners, if desired, to enhance taste.

Preparation Process

1. **Gather Ingredients**:

   - **Red Clover Powder**: 50%

   - **CoQ10 Powder**: 40%

   - **Binder**: 10% (e.g., cellulose powder or starch)

2. **Mixing**:

- In a clean, dry bowl, combine the red clover powder and CoQ10 powder thoroughly. Stir to ensure an even distribution of both powders.

- Gradually add the binder to the herb mixture, mixing well until the binder is fully incorporated. This helps the tablet mixture hold together effectively.

3. **Forming Tablets**:

- Use a tablet press or manual tablet-making tool to compress the herb mixture into tablets. Ensure that the tablets are uniform in size and adequately compressed to maintain their shape and effectiveness.

4. **Drying**:

- Allow the tablets to air dry completely on a clean, dry surface. Proper drying prevents moisture from affecting the tablets and ensures their stability.

5. **Storage**:

- Store the dried tablets in airtight containers to protect them from moisture, light, and air. Keep the containers in a cool, dry place to maintain the potency and extend the shelf life of the tablets.

- Label the containers with the preparation date and contents for easy identification.

Dosage and Usage

- **Recommended Dosage**: Typically, 1-2 tablets per day. Dosage may vary based on individual health needs and tablet potency. Consult with a healthcare provider for personalized dosage recommendations.

- **Usage Instructions**: Take the tablets with a glass of water. They can be consumed with meals or as needed to support hormonal balance, cardiovascular health, and energy levels.

Quality Control

- **Check for Uniformity**: Ensure that the tablets are consistently sized and weighted to provide accurate dosing and effectiveness.

- **Potency Testing**: Regularly test the tablets to confirm they contain the correct levels of active ingredients, ensuring they remain effective and safe for use.

Conclusion

Red clover and CoQ10 tablets offer a natural remedy to support hormonal balance, cardiovascular health, and overall energy levels. By combining the hormone-balancing and heart-supportive benefits of red clover with the cellular energy and antioxidant protection of CoQ10, these tablets provide a comprehensive approach to wellness. Following the preparation and storage guidelines will help maintain the tablets' potency and effectiveness, making them a valuable addition to a balanced health regimen.

For Skin Health

Calendula and Burdock Root Tablets

Calendula and burdock root are two herbs known for their skin-healing and detoxifying properties. Combining these herbs into tablets provides a natural remedy that supports skin health and overall detoxification. Calendula is celebrated for its soothing and anti-inflammatory effects, while burdock root is valued for its ability to purify the skin and support liver function.

Benefits of Calendula and Burdock Root

- **Calendula**: Calendula, also known as marigold, is renowned for its anti-inflammatory, antiseptic, and soothing properties. It is used to treat various skin conditions, including wounds, rashes, and irritation. Calendula promotes skin healing and helps reduce redness and inflammation.

- **Burdock Root**: Burdock root is traditionally used as a blood purifier and detoxifier. It helps clear toxins from the body and supports healthy skin by addressing issues like acne and eczema. Burdock root also contains antioxidants and essential nutrients that nourish the skin and promote overall wellness.

Ingredients

- **Calendula Powder**: Provides anti-inflammatory and skin-healing benefits.

- **Burdock Root Powder**: Supports detoxification and skin health.

- **Binder**: Such as cellulose powder or starch to ensure proper tablet formation.

- **Optional Additives**: Natural flavorings or sweeteners, if desired, to enhance taste.

Preparation Process

1. **Gather Ingredients**:

- **Calendula Powder**: 50%

- **Burdock Root Powder**: 40%

- **Binder**: 10% (e.g., cellulose powder or starch)

2. **Mixing**:

   - In a clean, dry bowl, combine the calendula powder and burdock root powder thoroughly. Stir to ensure even distribution of both powders.

   - Gradually add the binder to the herb mixture, mixing well until the binder is fully incorporated. This helps the tablet mixture hold together properly.

3. **Forming Tablets**:

   - Use a tablet press or manual tablet-making tool to compress the herb mixture into tablets. Ensure that the tablets are uniform in size and adequately compressed to maintain their shape and effectiveness.

4. **Drying**:

- Allow the tablets to air dry completely on a clean, dry surface. Proper drying prevents moisture from affecting the tablets and ensures their stability.

5. **Storage**:

- Store the dried tablets in airtight containers to protect them from moisture, light, and air. Keep the containers in a cool, dry place to maintain the potency and extend the shelf life of the tablets.

- Label the containers with the preparation date and contents for easy identification.

Dosage and Usage

- **Recommended Dosage**: Typically, 1-2 tablets per day. Dosage may vary based on individual health needs and tablet potency. Consult with a healthcare provider for personalized dosage recommendations.

- **Usage Instructions**: Take the tablets with a glass of water. They can be consumed with meals or as needed to support skin health and detoxification.

Quality Control

- **Check for Uniformity**: Ensure that the tablets are consistently sized and weighted for accurate dosing.

- **Potency Testing**: Regularly test the tablets to confirm they contain the correct levels of active ingredients, ensuring they remain effective and safe for use.

Conclusion

Calendula and burdock root tablets offer a natural remedy to support skin health and detoxification. By combining calendula's soothing and skin-healing properties with burdock root's detoxifying and skin-nourishing benefits, these tablets provide a comprehensive approach to promoting a healthy complexion and overall well-being. Following the preparation and storage guidelines ensures that the tablets retain their potency and effectiveness, making them a valuable addition to any health regimen.

Aloe Vera and Red Clover Tablets

Aloe vera and red clover are both valued for their health benefits, particularly for skin and hormonal balance. Combining these herbs into tablets offers a holistic approach to supporting skin health, hormonal equilibrium, and overall well-being. Aloe vera is renowned for its soothing and moisturizing properties, while red clover is known for its benefits to hormone balance and cardiovascular health.

Benefits of Aloe Vera and Red Clover

- **Aloe Vera**: Aloe vera is celebrated for its ability to soothe and moisturize the skin. It helps in healing wounds, reducing inflammation, and providing relief from various skin conditions. Aloe vera's internal use also supports digestive health and immune function.

- **Red Clover**: Red clover is rich in isoflavones, which have estrogen-like effects beneficial for hormonal balance. It can alleviate symptoms of menopause, support cardiovascular health, and improve skin elasticity. Red clover also has mild detoxifying properties that contribute to overall wellness.

Ingredients

- **Aloe Vera Powder**: Provides soothing, moisturizing, and healing benefits.

- **Red Clover Powder**: Supports hormonal balance and cardiovascular health.

- **Binder**: Such as cellulose powder or starch to help form tablets.

- **Optional Additives**: Natural flavorings or sweeteners, if desired, to enhance taste.

Preparation Process

1. **Gather Ingredients**:

   - **Aloe Vera Powder**: 50%

   - **Red Clover Powder**: 40%

   - **Binder**: 10% (e.g., cellulose powder or starch)

2. **Mixing**:

   - In a clean, dry bowl, combine the aloe vera powder and red clover powder thoroughly. Stir to ensure even distribution of both powders.

   - Gradually add the binder to the herb mixture and mix well until fully incorporated. This helps the tablet mixture hold together properly.

3. **Forming Tablets**:

   - Use a tablet press or manual tablet-making tool to compress the herb mixture into tablets. Ensure that the tablets are uniform in size and adequately compressed to maintain their shape and effectiveness.

4. **Drying**:

   o Allow the tablets to air dry completely on a clean, dry surface. Proper drying prevents moisture from affecting the tablets and ensures their stability.

5. **Storage**:

   o Store the dried tablets in airtight containers to protect them from moisture, light, and air. Keep the containers in a cool, dry place to maintain the potency and extend the shelf life of the tablets.

   o Label the containers with the preparation date and contents for easy identification.

Dosage and Usage

- **Recommended Dosage**: Typically, 1-2 tablets per day. Dosage may vary based on individual health needs and tablet potency. Consult with a healthcare provider for personalized dosage recommendations.

- **Usage Instructions**: Take the tablets with a glass of water. They can be consumed with meals or as needed to support skin health, hormonal balance, and overall wellness.

Quality Control

- **Check for Uniformity**: Ensure that the tablets are consistently sized and weighted for accurate dosing.

- **Potency Testing**: Regularly test the tablets to confirm they contain the correct levels of active ingredients, ensuring they remain effective and safe.

Conclusion

Aloe vera and red clover tablets offer a natural remedy to support skin health, hormonal balance, and overall well-being. By combining the soothing and healing properties of aloe vera with the hormonal support and cardiovascular benefits of red clover, these tablets provide a comprehensive approach to maintaining health and wellness. Following the preparation and storage guidelines ensures that the tablets retain their potency and effectiveness, making them a valuable addition to a health regimen.

Neem and Green Tea Tablets

Neem and green tea are renowned for their potent health benefits, particularly in supporting skin health and overall wellness. Combining these two herbs into tablets provides a powerful natural remedy with antioxidant, anti-inflammatory, and detoxifying properties. Neem is well-known for its cleansing and skin-soothing effects, while green tea offers significant antioxidant and metabolism-boosting benefits.

Benefits of Neem and Green Tea

- **Neem**: Neem is celebrated for its anti-inflammatory, antibacterial, and antifungal properties. It is widely used for treating various skin conditions such as acne, eczema, and psoriasis. Neem also supports detoxification and can help improve overall skin health by clearing impurities from the body.

- **Green Tea**: Green tea is rich in antioxidants, particularly catechins, which help protect cells from oxidative stress and support overall health. It has anti-inflammatory properties, boosts metabolism, and can improve skin appearance by reducing redness and promoting a healthy complexion.

Ingredients

- **Neem Powder**: Provides anti-inflammatory, antibacterial, and detoxifying benefits.

- **Green Tea Powder**: Offers antioxidant protection, supports metabolism, and enhances skin health.

- **Binder**: Such as cellulose powder or starch to ensure proper tablet formation.

- **Optional Additives**: Natural flavorings or sweeteners, if desired, to enhance taste.

Preparation Process

1. **Gather Ingredients**:

   - **Neem Powder**: 50%

   - **Green Tea Powder**: 40%

   - **Binder**: 10% (e.g., cellulose powder or starch)

2. **Mixing**:

   - In a clean, dry bowl, combine the neem powder and green tea powder thoroughly. Stir to ensure an even distribution of both powders.

- Gradually add the binder to the herb mixture and mix well until fully incorporated. This helps the tablet mixture hold together properly.

3. **Forming Tablets**:

- Use a tablet press or manual tablet-making tool to compress the herb mixture into tablets. Ensure that the tablets are uniform in size and adequately compressed to maintain their shape and effectiveness.

4. **Drying**:

- Allow the tablets to air dry completely on a clean, dry surface. Proper drying prevents moisture from affecting the tablets and ensures their stability.

5. **Storage**:

- Store the dried tablets in airtight containers to protect them from moisture, light, and air. Keep the containers in a cool, dry place to maintain potency and extend shelf life.

- Label the containers with the preparation date and contents for easy identification.

Dosage and Usage

- **Recommended Dosage**: Typically, 1-2 tablets per day. Dosage may vary based on individual health needs and tablet potency. Consult with a healthcare provider for personalized dosage recommendations.

- **Usage Instructions**: Take the tablets with a glass of water. They can be consumed with meals or as needed to support skin health, detoxification, and overall wellness.

Quality Control

- **Check for Uniformity**: Ensure that the tablets are consistently sized and weighted for accurate dosing.

- **Potency Testing**: Regularly test the tablets to confirm they contain the correct levels of active ingredients, ensuring they remain effective and safe.

Conclusion

Neem and green tea tablets offer a natural remedy to support skin health, detoxification, and overall wellness. By combining neem's cleansing and skin-soothing properties with green tea's antioxidant and metabolism-boosting benefits, these tablets provide a comprehensive approach to maintaining health. Following the preparation and storage guidelines ensures that the tablets retain their potency and effectiveness, making them a valuable addition to any health regimen.

Comfrey and Gotu Kola Tablets

Comfrey and gotu kola are both well-regarded for their therapeutic properties, particularly in promoting tissue repair and improving skin health. Combining these two herbs into tablets creates a potent remedy that supports healing, reduces inflammation, and enhances overall skin vitality. Comfrey is known for its cell-regenerating abilities, while gotu kola is valued for its role in collagen production and skin elasticity.

Benefits of Comfrey and Gotu Kola

- **Comfrey**: Comfrey is known for its high content of allantoin, a compound that promotes cell regeneration and healing. It is traditionally used to support the repair of damaged tissues, reduce inflammation, and treat wounds and bruises. Comfrey's application in herbal medicine is particularly focused on its external uses, but its benefits can extend internally as well.

- **Gotu Kola**: Gotu kola is revered for its ability to enhance collagen production and improve skin elasticity. It supports wound healing, reduces the appearance of scars, and promotes healthy circulation. Gotu kola is also beneficial for mental clarity and cognitive function, making it a versatile herb for overall wellness.

Ingredients

- **Comfrey Powder**: Provides cell-regenerating and anti-inflammatory benefits.

- **Gotu Kola Powder**: Supports collagen production, skin elasticity, and overall skin health.

- **Binder**: Such as cellulose powder or starch to ensure proper tablet formation.

- **Optional Additives**: Natural flavorings or sweeteners, if desired, to enhance taste.

Preparation Process

1. **Gather Ingredients**:

   - **Comfrey Powder**: 50%

   - **Gotu Kola Powder**: 40%

- **Binder**: 10% (e.g., cellulose powder or starch)

2. **Mixing**:

   - In a clean, dry bowl, combine the comfrey powder and gotu kola powder thoroughly. Stir to ensure even distribution of both powders.

   - Gradually add the binder to the herb mixture and mix well until fully incorporated. This helps the tablet mixture hold together properly.

3. **Forming Tablets**:

   - Use a tablet press or manual tablet-making tool to compress the herb mixture into tablets. Ensure that the tablets are uniform in size and adequately compressed to maintain their shape and effectiveness.

4. **Drying**:

   - Allow the tablets to air dry completely on a clean, dry surface. Proper drying prevents moisture from affecting the tablets and ensures their stability.

5. **Storage**:

- Store the dried tablets in airtight containers to protect them from moisture, light, and air. Keep the containers in a cool, dry place to maintain potency and extend shelf life.

- Label the containers with the preparation date and contents for easy identification.

Dosage and Usage

- **Recommended Dosage**: Typically, 1-2 tablets per day. Dosage may vary based on individual health needs and tablet potency. Consult with a healthcare provider for personalized dosage recommendations.

- **Usage Instructions**: Take the tablets with a glass of water. They can be consumed with meals or as needed to support skin health, tissue repair, and overall wellness.

Quality Control

- **Check for Uniformity**: Ensure that the tablets are consistently sized and weighted for accurate dosing.

- **Potency Testing**: Regularly test the tablets to confirm they contain the correct levels of active ingredients, ensuring they remain effective and safe.

Conclusion

Comfrey and gotu kola tablets offer a natural remedy to support tissue repair, reduce inflammation, and enhance skin health. By combining comfrey's cell-regenerating properties with gotu kola's collagen-boosting and skin-elasticity benefits, these tablets provide a comprehensive approach to maintaining and improving skin vitality and overall wellness. Following the preparation and storage guidelines ensures that the tablets retain their potency and effectiveness, making them a valuable addition to any health regimen.

For Hormonal Balance

Vitex and Dong Quai Tablets

Vitex (Chaste Tree) and Dong Quai are both powerful herbs known for their beneficial effects on hormonal balance, particularly in supporting the female reproductive system. Combining these herbs into tablets creates a synergistic formula designed to address a range of hormonal issues, including menstrual irregularities, menopausal symptoms, and overall reproductive health.

Benefits of Vitex and Dong Quai

- **Vitex (Chaste Tree)**: Vitex is widely used to balance hormones by influencing the pituitary gland, which regulates the production of estrogen and progesterone. It is particularly helpful for managing symptoms of premenstrual syndrome (PMS), irregular menstrual cycles, and menopausal discomfort. Vitex helps promote regular menstruation and supports overall reproductive health.

- **Dong Quai**: Known as the "female ginseng," Dong Quai is used to support the female reproductive system and address menstrual and menopausal symptoms. It helps improve blood circulation and is believed to aid in hormone regulation and balance. Dong Quai is also traditionally used to relieve menstrual cramps and support overall vitality.

Ingredients

- **Vitex Powder**: 50%

- **Dong Quai Powder**: 40%

- **Binder**: 10% (e.g., cellulose powder or starch)

Preparation Process

1. **Gather Ingredients**:

   - **Vitex Powder**: 50%

   - **Dong Quai Powder**: 40%

- **Binder**: 10% (e.g., cellulose powder or starch)

2. **Mixing**:

   - In a clean, dry bowl, thoroughly combine the Vitex powder and Dong Quai powder. Ensure an even distribution of both powders.

   - Gradually add the binder to the herb mixture and mix well until fully incorporated. This helps the tablet mixture hold together properly.

3. **Forming Tablets**:

   - Use a tablet press or manual tablet-making tool to compress the herb mixture into tablets. Ensure that the tablets are uniform in size and adequately compressed to maintain their shape and effectiveness.

4. **Drying**:

   - Allow the tablets to air dry completely on a clean, dry surface. Proper drying prevents moisture from affecting the tablets and ensures their stability.

5. **Storage**:

- Store the dried tablets in airtight containers to protect them from moisture, light, and air. Keep the containers in a cool, dry place to maintain potency and extend shelf life.

- Label the containers with the preparation date and contents for easy identification.

Dosage and Usage

- **Recommended Dosage**: Typically, 1-2 tablets per day. Dosage may vary based on individual health needs and tablet potency. Consult with a healthcare provider for personalized dosage recommendations.

- **Usage Instructions**: Take the tablets with a glass of water. They can be consumed with meals or as needed to support hormonal balance and reproductive health.

Quality Control

- **Check for Uniformity**: Ensure that the tablets are consistently sized and weighted for accurate dosing.

- **Potency Testing**: Regularly test the tablets to confirm they contain the correct levels of active ingredients, ensuring they remain effective and safe.

Conclusion

Vitex and Dong Quai tablets offer a natural remedy to support hormonal balance and overall reproductive health. By combining Vitex's hormone-regulating properties with Dong Quai's circulatory and vitality-enhancing benefits, these tablets provide a comprehensive approach to managing menstrual irregularities, menopausal symptoms, and overall hormonal well-being. Following the preparation and storage guidelines ensures that the tablets retain their potency and effectiveness, making them a valuable addition to any health regimen focused on hormonal balance.

Black Cohosh and Evening Primrose Tablets

Black Cohosh and Evening Primrose are two well-regarded herbs known for their support in managing menopausal symptoms and promoting overall hormonal health. Combining these herbs into tablets creates a potent remedy aimed at alleviating common issues associated with menopause and supporting hormonal balance.

Benefits of Black Cohosh and Evening Primrose

- **Black Cohosh**: Black Cohosh is widely used for managing symptoms of menopause, such as hot flashes, night sweats, and mood swings. It works by influencing estrogen receptors in the body, which helps to reduce the intensity of menopausal symptoms. Black Cohosh is also known for its anti-inflammatory properties and its ability to support reproductive health.

- **Evening Primrose**: Evening Primrose Oil is rich in gamma-linolenic acid (GLA), a type of essential fatty acid that supports hormonal balance. It is particularly beneficial for alleviating symptoms of premenstrual syndrome (PMS) and menopause, such as mood swings and breast tenderness. Evening Primrose Oil also supports skin health and overall well-being.

Ingredients

- **Black Cohosh Powder**: 50%

- **Evening Primrose Oil Powder**: 40%

- **Binder**: 10% (e.g., cellulose powder or starch)

Preparation Process

1. **Gather Ingredients**:

   ○ **Black Cohosh Powder**: 50%

   ○ **Evening Primrose Oil Powder**: 40%

- o **Binder**: 10% (e.g., cellulose powder or starch)

2. **Mixing**:

   - o In a clean, dry bowl, combine the Black Cohosh powder and Evening Primrose Oil powder thoroughly. Stir to ensure an even distribution of both powders.

   - o Gradually add the binder to the herb mixture and mix well until fully incorporated. This ensures that the tablet mixture holds together properly.

3. **Forming Tablets**:

   - o Use a tablet press or manual tablet-making tool to compress the herb mixture into tablets. Ensure that the tablets are uniform in size and adequately compressed to maintain their shape and effectiveness.

4. **Drying**:

   - o Allow the tablets to air dry completely on a clean, dry surface. Proper drying prevents moisture from affecting the tablets and ensures their stability.

5. **Storage**:

○ Store the dried tablets in airtight containers to protect them from moisture, light, and air. Keep the containers in a cool, dry place to maintain potency and extend shelf life.

○ Label the containers with the preparation date and contents for easy identification.

Dosage and Usage

- **Recommended Dosage**: Typically, 1-2 tablets per day. Dosage may vary based on individual health needs and tablet potency. Consult with a healthcare provider for personalized dosage recommendations.

- **Usage Instructions**: Take the tablets with a glass of water. They can be consumed with meals or as needed to support hormonal balance and alleviate menopausal symptoms.

Quality Control

- **Check for Uniformity**: Ensure that the tablets are consistently sized and weighted for accurate dosing.

- **Potency Testing**: Regularly test the tablets to confirm they contain the correct levels of active ingredients, ensuring they remain effective and safe.

Conclusion

Black Cohosh and Evening Primrose tablets offer a natural remedy to support hormonal balance and manage menopausal symptoms. By combining Black Cohosh's ability to alleviate hot flashes and mood swings with Evening Primrose Oil's hormone-regulating and skin-supporting benefits, these tablets provide a comprehensive approach to managing menopause and supporting overall well-being. Following the preparation and storage guidelines ensures that the tablets retain their potency and effectiveness, making them a valuable addition to any health regimen focused on hormonal health and menopause management.

Shatavari and Maca Root Tablets

Shatavari and Maca Root are two herbs renowned for their ability to support reproductive health and hormonal balance. Combining these herbs into tablets creates a powerful formulation aimed at enhancing vitality, managing hormonal fluctuations, and supporting overall well-being.

Benefits of Shatavari and Maca Root

- **Shatavari**: Shatavari is a revered adaptogen in Ayurvedic medicine known for its supportive role in female reproductive health. It helps balance hormones, alleviate symptoms of PMS and menopause, and promote overall vitality. Shatavari also supports digestive health and enhances the body's ability to cope with stress.

- **Maca Root**: Maca Root is a well-known adaptogen that boosts energy levels and supports hormonal balance. It is often used to enhance stamina, improve mood, and support reproductive health. Maca is beneficial for both men and women and helps address symptoms related to hormonal imbalances, such as fatigue and mood swings.

Ingredients

- **Shatavari Powder**: 50%

- **Maca Root Powder**: 40%

- **Binder**: 10% (e.g., cellulose powder or starch)

Preparation Process

1. **Gather Ingredients**:

   - **Shatavari Powder**: 50%

   - **Maca Root Powder**: 40%

   - **Binder**: 10% (e.g., cellulose powder or starch)

2. **Mixing**:

   ○ In a clean, dry bowl, combine the Shatavari powder and Maca Root powder thoroughly. Stir to ensure an even distribution of both powders.

   ○ Gradually add the binder to the herb mixture and mix well until fully incorporated. This helps the tablet mixture hold together properly.

3. **Forming Tablets**:

   ○ Use a tablet press or manual tablet-making tool to compress the herb mixture into tablets. Ensure that the tablets are uniform in size and adequately compressed to maintain their shape and effectiveness.

4. **Drying**:

   ○ Allow the tablets to air dry completely on a clean, dry surface. Proper drying prevents moisture from affecting the tablets and ensures their stability.

5. **Storage**:

○ Store the dried tablets in airtight containers to protect them from moisture, light, and air. Keep the containers in a cool, dry place to maintain potency and extend shelf life.

○ Label the containers with the preparation date and contents for easy identification.

Dosage and Usage

- **Recommended Dosage**: Typically, 1-2 tablets per day. Dosage may vary based on individual health needs and tablet potency. Consult with a healthcare provider for personalized dosage recommendations.

- **Usage Instructions**: Take the tablets with a glass of water. They can be consumed with meals or as needed to support hormonal balance and overall vitality.

Quality Control

- **Check for Uniformity**: Ensure that the tablets are consistently sized and weighted for accurate dosing.

- **Potency Testing**: Regularly test the tablets to confirm they contain the correct levels of active ingredients, ensuring they remain effective and safe.

Conclusion

Shatavari and Maca Root tablets offer a natural and effective approach to supporting hormonal balance and enhancing overall vitality. By combining Shatavari's benefits for reproductive health and stress management with Maca Root's energy-boosting and hormone-regulating properties, these tablets provide a holistic solution for addressing hormonal fluctuations and promoting well-being. Following the preparation and storage guidelines ensures that the tablets retain their potency and effectiveness, making them a valuable addition to any health regimen focused on reproductive and hormonal health.

Tribulus Terrestris and Soy Isoflavones Tablets

Tribulus Terrestris and Soy Isoflavones are two powerful ingredients used to support hormonal balance and enhance overall health. Combining these herbs into tablets creates a formulation designed to improve vitality, support reproductive health, and address various hormonal issues.

Benefits of Tribulus Terrestris and Soy Isoflavones

- **Tribulus Terrestris**: Tribulus Terrestris is a traditional herb used for its potential benefits in enhancing libido, supporting male reproductive health, and boosting overall vitality. It is believed to improve testosterone levels, which can aid in increasing energy, stamina, and muscle mass. Additionally, Tribulus may support cardiovascular health and reduce symptoms of hormonal imbalance.

- **Soy Isoflavones**: Soy Isoflavones are plant compounds found in soybeans that mimic the effects of estrogen in the body. They are used to support hormonal balance, alleviate menopausal symptoms, and promote bone health. Soy Isoflavones are also known for their antioxidant properties, which help protect cells from damage and support overall health.

Ingredients

- **Tribulus Terrestris Powder**: 50%

- **Soy Isoflavones Powder**: 40%

- **Binder**: 10% (e.g., cellulose powder or starch)

Preparation Process

1. **Gather Ingredients**:

     - **Tribulus Terrestris Powder**: 50%

     - **Soy Isoflavones Powder**: 40%

- Binder: 10% (e.g., cellulose powder or starch)

2. **Mixing**:

   - In a clean, dry bowl, thoroughly combine the Tribulus Terrestris powder and Soy Isoflavones powder. Stir to ensure an even distribution of both powders.

   - Gradually add the binder to the herb mixture and mix well until fully incorporated. This helps the tablet mixture hold together properly.

3. **Forming Tablets**:

   - Use a tablet press or manual tablet-making tool to compress the herb mixture into tablets. Ensure that the tablets are uniform in size and adequately compressed to maintain their shape and effectiveness.

4. **Drying**:

   - Allow the tablets to air dry completely on a clean, dry surface. Proper drying prevents moisture from affecting the tablets and ensures their stability.

5. **Storage**:

- Store the dried tablets in airtight containers to protect them from moisture, light, and air. Keep the containers in a cool, dry place to maintain potency and extend shelf life.

- Label the containers with the preparation date and contents for easy identification.

Dosage and Usage

- **Recommended Dosage**: Typically, 1-2 tablets per day. Dosage may vary based on individual health needs and tablet potency. Consult with a healthcare provider for personalized dosage recommendations.

- **Usage Instructions**: Take the tablets with a glass of water. They can be consumed with meals or as needed to support hormonal balance and overall vitality.

Quality Control

- **Check for Uniformity**: Ensure that the tablets are consistently sized and weighted for accurate dosing.

- **Potency Testing**: Regularly test the tablets to confirm they contain the correct levels of active ingredients, ensuring they remain effective and safe.

Conclusion

Tribulus Terrestris and Soy Isoflavones tablets provide a natural approach to enhancing vitality and supporting hormonal balance. By combining Tribulus's benefits for reproductive health and energy with Soy Isoflavones' estrogen-mimicking properties, these tablets offer a comprehensive solution for managing hormonal fluctuations and improving overall well-being. Adhering to the preparation and storage guidelines ensures that the tablets maintain their potency and effectiveness, making them a valuable addition to any health regimen focused on hormonal health and vitality.

For Cognitive Function

Ginkgo Biloba and Bacopa Tablets

Ginkgo Biloba and Bacopa are two powerful herbs known for their cognitive-enhancing properties. Combining these herbs into tablets creates a formulation designed to improve memory, focus, and overall cognitive function. This blend supports brain health by promoting better circulation, reducing mental fatigue, and enhancing mental clarity.

Benefits of Ginkgo Biloba and Bacopa

- **Ginkgo Biloba**: Ginkgo Biloba is well-known for its ability to improve blood flow to the brain, which enhances memory and cognitive function. It has antioxidant properties that protect brain cells from oxidative stress and damage. Ginkgo is also used to improve concentration and mental clarity, making it a valuable herb for cognitive support.

- **Bacopa Monnieri**: Bacopa Monnieri is an adaptogen that supports cognitive health by improving memory, learning, and brain function. It helps enhance synaptic communication in the brain and promotes the growth of nerve cells. Bacopa is also effective in reducing stress and anxiety, which can further enhance cognitive performance.

Ingredients

- **Ginkgo Biloba Powder**: 50%

- **Bacopa Monnieri Powder**: 40%

- **Binder**: 10% (e.g., cellulose powder or starch)

Preparation Process

1. **Gather Ingredients**:

   - **Ginkgo Biloba Powder**: 50%

   - **Bacopa Monnieri Powder**: 40%

o **Binder**: 10% (e.g., cellulose powder or starch)

2. **Mixing**:

   o In a clean, dry bowl, thoroughly combine the Ginkgo Biloba powder and Bacopa Monnieri powder. Stir the mixture to ensure an even distribution of both powders.

   o Gradually add the binder to the herb mixture and mix well until fully incorporated. The binder helps the tablet mixture hold together.

3. **Forming Tablets**:

   o Use a tablet press or manual tablet-making tool to compress the herb mixture into tablets. Ensure that the tablets are uniform in size and adequately compressed to maintain their shape and effectiveness.

4. **Drying**:

   o Allow the tablets to air dry completely on a clean, dry surface. Proper drying is crucial to prevent moisture from affecting the tablets and to ensure their stability.

5. **Storage**:

- Store the dried tablets in airtight containers to protect them from moisture, light, and air. Keep the containers in a cool, dry place to maintain potency and extend shelf life.

- Label the containers with the preparation date and contents for easy identification.

Dosage and Usage

- **Recommended Dosage**: Typically, 1-2 tablets per day. Dosage may vary based on individual health needs and tablet potency. Consult with a healthcare provider for personalized dosage recommendations.

- **Usage Instructions**: Take the tablets with a glass of water. They can be consumed with meals or as needed to support cognitive function and mental clarity.

Quality Control

- **Check for Uniformity**: Ensure that the tablets are consistently sized and weighted for accurate dosing.

- **Potency Testing**: Regularly test the tablets to confirm they contain the correct levels of active ingredients, ensuring they remain effective and safe.

Conclusion

Ginkgo Biloba and Bacopa Tablets offer a natural solution for enhancing cognitive function and improving mental clarity. By combining the memory-boosting and circulation-enhancing properties of Ginkgo Biloba with the cognitive-supportive and stress-reducing benefits of Bacopa, these tablets provide a comprehensive approach to supporting brain health. Following the preparation and storage guidelines ensures that the tablets maintain their potency and effectiveness, making them a valuable addition to any regimen focused on cognitive enhancement.

Lion's Mane Mushroom and Rhodiola Tablets

Lion's Mane Mushroom and Rhodiola are two powerful herbs known for their cognitive and adaptogenic benefits. Combining these ingredients into tablets creates a formulation that supports brain health, enhances cognitive function, and helps manage stress.

Benefits of Lion's Mane Mushroom and Rhodiola

- **Lion's Mane Mushroom**: Lion's Mane is renowned for its neuroprotective properties and ability to enhance cognitive function. It promotes the growth and repair of nerve cells, which can support memory, concentration, and overall mental clarity. Lion's Mane is also known to reduce symptoms of anxiety and depression, contributing to improved mental well-being.

- **Rhodiola Rosea**: Rhodiola is an adaptogenic herb that helps the body adapt to stress and reduce mental fatigue. It supports cognitive function by enhancing mental clarity and focus. Rhodiola also helps improve mood and overall energy levels, making it a valuable herb for managing stress and supporting cognitive health.

Ingredients

- **Lion's Mane Mushroom Powder**: 50%
- **Rhodiola Rosea Powder**: 40%
- **Binder**: 10% (e.g., cellulose powder or starch)

Preparation Process

1. **Gather Ingredients**:

   o **Lion's Mane Mushroom Powder**: 50%

   o **Rhodiola Rosea Powder**: 40%

   o **Binder**: 10% (e.g., cellulose powder or starch)

2. **Mixing**:

   - Combine the Lion's Mane Mushroom powder and Rhodiola Rosea powder in a clean, dry bowl. Stir the mixture thoroughly to ensure an even distribution of both powders.

   - Gradually add the binder to the herb mixture and mix well until fully incorporated. The binder helps the tablet mixture hold together and maintain its shape.

3. **Forming Tablets**:

   - Use a tablet press or manual tablet-making tool to compress the herb mixture into tablets. Ensure that the tablets are uniform in size and adequately compressed to ensure consistency and effectiveness.

4. **Drying**:

   - Allow the tablets to air dry completely on a clean, dry surface. Proper drying is essential to prevent moisture from affecting the tablets and to ensure their stability.

5. **Storage**:

- Store the dried tablets in airtight containers to protect them from moisture, light, and air. Keep the containers in a cool, dry place to maintain potency and extend shelf life.

- Label the containers with the preparation date and contents for easy identification.

Dosage and Usage

- **Recommended Dosage**: Typically, 1-2 tablets per day. Dosage may vary based on individual health needs and tablet potency. Consult with a healthcare provider for personalized dosage recommendations.

- **Usage Instructions**: Take the tablets with a glass of water. They can be consumed with meals or as needed to support cognitive function and manage stress.

Quality Control

- **Check for Uniformity**: Ensure that the tablets are consistently sized and weighted for accurate dosing.

- **Potency Testing**: Regularly test the tablets to confirm they contain the correct levels of active ingredients, ensuring they remain effective and safe.

Conclusion

Lion's Mane Mushroom and Rhodiola Tablets offer a natural approach to enhancing cognitive function and managing stress. Combining Lion's Mane's neuroprotective benefits with Rhodiola's adaptogenic properties provides a comprehensive solution for improving mental clarity, reducing stress, and supporting overall cognitive health. Adhering to the preparation and storage guidelines ensures that the tablets maintain their potency and effectiveness, making them a valuable addition to any health regimen focused on cognitive enhancement and stress management.

Sage and Peppermint Tablets

Sage and Peppermint are herbs known for their benefits to digestive health and cognitive function. Combining these ingredients into tablets creates a formulation that supports gastrointestinal comfort, mental clarity, and overall well-being.

Benefits of Sage and Peppermint

- **Sage**: Sage is celebrated for its ability to support digestive health, reduce inflammation, and enhance cognitive function. It can help alleviate digestive issues such as bloating and indigestion, and its antioxidant properties contribute to overall health. Sage is also known for its cognitive benefits, including improved memory and mental clarity.

- **Peppermint**: Peppermint is widely used to ease digestive discomfort, including symptoms like gas, bloating, and nausea. Its antispasmodic properties help relax the digestive tract, making it useful for managing gastrointestinal issues. Additionally, peppermint has a refreshing effect and can enhance mental alertness and clarity.

Ingredients

- **Sage Powder**: 50%

- **Peppermint Powder**: 40%

- **Binder**: 10% (e.g., cellulose powder or starch)

Preparation Process

1. **Gather Ingredients**:

   - **Sage Powder**: 50%

   - **Peppermint Powder**: 40%

   - **Binder**: 10% (e.g., cellulose powder or starch)

2. **Mixing**:

   o In a clean, dry bowl, thoroughly combine the Sage powder and Peppermint powder. Stir the mixture to ensure an even distribution of both powders.

   o Gradually add the binder to the herb mixture and mix well until fully incorporated. The binder helps the tablet mixture maintain its shape and consistency.

3. **Forming Tablets**:

   o Use a tablet press or manual tablet-making tool to compress the herb mixture into tablets. Ensure that the tablets are uniform in size and adequately compressed to ensure consistency and effectiveness.

4. **Drying**:

   o Allow the tablets to air dry completely on a clean, dry surface. Proper drying is essential to prevent moisture from affecting the tablets and to ensure their stability.

5. **Storage**:

- Store the dried tablets in airtight containers to protect them from moisture, light, and air. Keep the containers in a cool, dry place to maintain potency and extend shelf life.

- Label the containers with the preparation date and contents for easy identification.

Dosage and Usage

- **Recommended Dosage**: Typically, 1-2 tablets per day. Dosage may vary based on individual health needs and tablet potency. Consult with a healthcare provider for personalized dosage recommendations.

- **Usage Instructions**: Take the tablets with a glass of water. They can be consumed with meals or as needed to support digestive health and mental clarity.

Quality Control

- **Check for Uniformity**: Ensure that the tablets are consistently sized and weighted for accurate dosing.

- **Potency Testing**: Regularly test the tablets to confirm they contain the correct levels of active ingredients, ensuring they remain effective and safe.

Conclusion

Sage and Peppermint Tablets provide a natural solution for supporting digestive health and enhancing cognitive function. The combination of Sage's digestive and cognitive benefits with Peppermint's soothing properties creates a balanced formulation that promotes overall well-being. Following the preparation and storage guidelines ensures that the tablets maintain their potency and effectiveness, making them a valuable addition to any health regimen focused on digestive comfort and mental clarity.

Ashwagandha and Schisandra Tablets

Ashwagandha and Schisandra are powerful adaptogenic herbs known for their stress-relieving and overall health-promoting properties. Combining these herbs into tablets creates a formulation designed to support stress management, enhance energy levels, and improve overall vitality.

Benefits of Ashwagandha and Schisandra

- **Ashwagandha**: Ashwagandha, also known as Withania somnifera, is an adaptogen that helps the body cope with stress and anxiety. It is known for its ability to improve stamina, reduce cortisol levels, and support mental clarity. Ashwagandha also contributes to overall well-being by enhancing energy levels, supporting immune function, and promoting a balanced mood.

- **Schisandra**: Schisandra, or Schisandra chinensis, is a potent adaptogen that supports the body's response to stress and enhances endurance. It is known for its ability to improve mental performance, boost liver function, and increase overall vitality. Schisandra also helps to stabilize mood and improve resistance to physical and emotional stress.

Ingredients

- **Ashwagandha Powder**: 50%

- **Schisandra Powder**: 40%

- **Binder**: 10% (e.g., cellulose powder or starch)

Preparation Process

1. **Gather Ingredients**:

   - **Ashwagandha Powder**: 50%

   - **Schisandra Powder**: 40%

   - **Binder**: 10% (e.g., cellulose powder or starch)

2. **Mixing**:

- In a clean, dry bowl, combine the Ashwagandha powder and Schisandra powder. Stir thoroughly to ensure an even distribution of both powders.

- Gradually add the binder to the herb mixture and mix well until fully incorporated. The binder helps the tablet mixture hold together and maintain its shape.

3. **Forming Tablets**:

- Use a tablet press or manual tablet-making tool to compress the herb mixture into tablets. Ensure that the tablets are uniform in size and adequately compressed to ensure consistency and effectiveness.

4. **Drying**:

- Allow the tablets to air dry completely on a clean, dry surface. Proper drying is essential to prevent moisture from affecting the tablets and to ensure their stability.

5. **Storage**:

- Store the dried tablets in airtight containers to protect them from moisture, light, and air. Keep the containers in a cool, dry place to maintain potency and extend shelf life.

- Label the containers with the preparation date and contents for easy identification.

Dosage and Usage

- **Recommended Dosage**: Typically, 1-2 tablets per day. Dosage may vary based on individual health needs and tablet potency. Consult with a healthcare provider for personalized dosage recommendations.

- **Usage Instructions**: Take the tablets with a glass of water. They can be consumed with meals or as needed to support stress management and overall vitality.

Quality Control

- **Check for Uniformity**: Ensure that the tablets are consistently sized and weighted for accurate dosing.

- **Potency Testing**: Regularly test the tablets to confirm they contain the correct levels of active ingredients, ensuring they remain effective and safe.

Conclusion

Ashwagandha and Schisandra Tablets offer a natural solution for managing stress and enhancing overall vitality. Combining Ashwagandha's stress-relief and energy-boosting properties with Schisandra's adaptogenic benefits provides a comprehensive approach to improving resilience and well-being. Adhering to the preparation and storage guidelines ensures that the tablets maintain their potency and effectiveness, making them a valuable addition to any health regimen focused on stress management and vitality.

Chapter 6: Advanced Techniques and Tips

Customizing Your Herbal Tablet Formulations

Customizing herbal tablet formulations allows you to tailor your products to specific health needs, preferences, and therapeutic goals. This process involves selecting and blending herbs, adjusting dosages, and creating unique formulations that address individual health concerns or desired outcomes. Here's how to effectively customize your herbal tablet formulations:

Identifying Health Goals and Needs

1. **Define Objectives**: Determine the specific health benefits you want your herbal tablets to provide. This could include supporting immune health, enhancing cognitive function, alleviating stress, or addressing digestive issues.

2. **Research Herbal Properties**: Investigate the properties and benefits of various herbs to find those that align with your health goals. Look for herbs with proven efficacy and complementary actions to create a balanced and effective formulation.

3. **Consult Expertise**: Seek advice from herbalists, naturopaths, or healthcare professionals to ensure your formulations are safe and

effective. They can provide insights into the best herb combinations and dosages for your intended outcomes.

Selecting and Blending Herbs

1. **Choose Key Herbs**: Select herbs known for their effectiveness in achieving your health goals. Consider herbs with synergistic effects that enhance each other's benefits. For example, combining adaptogens like Ashwagandha with calming herbs like Chamomile can create a balanced stress-relief formula.

2. **Consider Herb Interactions**: Be mindful of how different herbs interact with each other. Some herbs may enhance the effects of others, while others may counteract or diminish their benefits. Understanding these interactions helps in creating a well-rounded formulation.

3. **Blend Ratios**: Adjust the ratios of each herb based on their potency and desired effects. Higher doses of certain herbs may be necessary for more pronounced effects, while others may need to be used in smaller amounts to avoid potential side effects.

Formulating for Specific Conditions

1. **Immune Support**: For immune-boosting tablets, consider combining herbs like Echinacea and Elderberry, which are known for their antiviral and immune-enhancing properties. You may also include adaptogens like Astragalus to support overall immune resilience.

2. **Digestive Health**: To support digestive health, blend herbs like Peppermint and Ginger for their soothing effects on the gastrointestinal tract. Incorporate herbs like Fennel and Slippery Elm for additional digestive support and anti-inflammatory benefits.

3. **Stress and Anxiety**: Create a stress-relief formulation by combining calming herbs such as Ashwagandha and Valerian Root. You might also add adaptogens like Rhodiola to enhance the body's ability to cope with stress.

Adjusting Dosages and Potency

1. **Determine Dosage**: Research the recommended dosages for each herb to ensure effectiveness and safety. Dosages can vary based on factors such as age, health condition, and individual response.

2. **Test and Adjust**: Start with standard dosages and test the effectiveness of your tablets. Based on user feedback or clinical trials, adjust the herb ratios and dosages to improve potency and achieve desired outcomes.

3. **Monitor Side Effects**: Pay attention to any potential side effects or interactions, especially when combining multiple herbs. Adjust formulations as needed to minimize adverse effects and enhance safety.

Creating Combination Formulas

1. **Balanced Blends**: Create combination formulas that address multiple health aspects in one tablet. For example, a tablet designed for overall wellness might include a mix of adaptogens, antioxidants, and digestive aids.

2. **Layered Benefits**: Develop layered benefits by combining herbs with different actions. For instance, a formulation for cognitive support might include memory-enhancing herbs like Ginkgo Biloba alongside stress-reducing herbs like Rhodiola.

3. **Personalization**: Offer customization options for users who may have specific needs or preferences. Allowing users to choose from a range of formulations or adjust dosages can cater to individual health goals.

Ensuring Quality and Consistency

1. **Standardize Ingredients**: Use standardized herbal extracts to ensure consistent potency and quality. This helps maintain uniformity in your

tablet formulations and ensures that each batch meets the desired specifications.

2. **Thorough Mixing**: Ensure that herbs and binders are thoroughly mixed to achieve uniform distribution of ingredients in each tablet. Inconsistent mixing can lead to variations in potency and effectiveness.

3. **Quality Control**: Implement strict quality control measures to monitor the consistency and effectiveness of your tablets. Regular testing and inspections can help maintain high standards and ensure the safety of your products.

Conclusion

Customizing your herbal tablet formulations allows you to create products that meet specific health needs and preferences. By carefully selecting and blending herbs, adjusting dosages, and ensuring quality and consistency, you can develop effective and targeted herbal tablets that provide meaningful health benefits. This approach not only enhances the effectiveness of your products but also ensures that they align with your goals and the needs of your users.

Combining Herbs for Enhanced Effects

Combining herbs, also known as herbal synergy, involves blending different herbs to create formulations that are more effective than using a single herb alone. This practice leverages the unique properties of each herb to enhance their collective benefits, targeting specific health conditions or overall wellness. Understanding how to combine herbs effectively can significantly boost the potency and therapeutic effects of your herbal tablets.

Understanding Herbal Synergy

- **Synergistic Effects**: Some herbs work synergistically, meaning their combined effects are greater than the sum of their individual effects. For example, pairing Echinacea with Elderberry can enhance immune support because these herbs boost immune function in complementary ways.

- **Complementary Actions**: Combining herbs with complementary actions can provide a balanced approach to addressing health concerns. For instance, pairing a calming herb like Valerian Root with an adaptogen like Ashwagandha can provide both relaxation and stress resilience, addressing both immediate symptoms and underlying causes of anxiety.

- **Herbal Potentiation**: This involves using certain herbs to enhance the absorption or effectiveness of other herbs. For example, black pepper contains piperine, which can increase the bioavailability of curcumin from turmeric, making the combination more effective for anti-inflammatory purposes.

Key Principles for Combining Herbs

- **Safety and Compatibility**: Ensure that the herbs you combine are safe to use together and do not have any adverse interactions. Some herbs can potentiate the effects of others, which may lead to stronger results or, in some cases, unwanted side effects.

- **Balanced Formulations**: Strive for balance in your formulations by combining herbs with different actions. For example, in a formulation for digestive health, you might combine soothing herbs like Slippery Elm with carminatives like Fennel to cover a broader range of digestive issues.

- **Targeted Benefits**: Focus on the specific health benefits you want to achieve with your herbal combination. Select herbs that target different aspects of the same condition, such as inflammation and pain, to create a more comprehensive remedy.

Examples of Effective Herbal Combinations

1. **Immune System Boosters**:

   o **Echinacea and Elderberry**: Echinacea stimulates the immune system, while Elderberry provides antiviral benefits. Together, they can enhance immune response and protect against infections.

   o **Astragalus and Ginger**: Astragalus is known for its immune-boosting properties, and Ginger is an anti-inflammatory and antioxidant. This combination supports overall immune health and helps reduce inflammation.

2. **Digestive Health Blends**:

   o **Peppermint and Ginger**: Both herbs soothe the digestive tract, reduce nausea, and relieve indigestion. This combination is excellent for general digestive support.

   o **Dandelion and Licorice Root**: Dandelion supports liver function and detoxification, while Licorice Root soothes mucous membranes and reduces inflammation in the digestive tract.

3. **Stress and Anxiety Relief**:

- **Chamomile and Lemon Balm**: Both herbs have calming effects on the nervous system and help reduce anxiety. Combining them can enhance relaxation and improve sleep quality.

- **Ashwagandha and Valerian Root**: Ashwagandha is an adaptogen that helps the body cope with stress, while Valerian Root is a sedative that helps promote relaxation and sleep.

4. **Pain and Inflammation Relief**:

- **Turmeric and Boswellia**: Turmeric contains curcumin, a powerful anti-inflammatory, while Boswellia (Frankincense) helps reduce joint inflammation and pain. This combination is particularly effective for conditions like arthritis.

- **Willow Bark and Arnica**: Willow Bark is a natural source of salicin, which helps reduce pain and inflammation, and Arnica is known for its anti-inflammatory properties, making this a powerful duo for managing pain.

5. **Cognitive Support and Enhancement**:

- **Ginkgo Biloba and Bacopa**: Ginkgo improves circulation and oxygenation to the brain, enhancing cognitive function, while

Bacopa is known for its memory-enhancing properties. Together, they provide comprehensive support for cognitive health.

- ○ **Lion's Mane Mushroom and Rhodiola**: Lion's Mane supports nerve regeneration and brain health, while Rhodiola is an adaptogen that improves mental clarity and reduces fatigue.

Formulation Strategies for Enhanced Effects

- **Layering Herbal Actions**: Combine herbs that provide immediate relief with those that offer long-term support. For example, in a formulation for joint pain, include fast-acting herbs like White Willow Bark with longer-acting herbs like Turmeric for sustained anti-inflammatory effects.

- **Balancing Potency and Gentle Herbs**: Combine potent herbs that have strong therapeutic effects with milder herbs that support overall health. This approach helps balance strong actions while minimizing potential side effects.

- **Optimizing Absorption**: Use herbs that enhance the absorption of others. For example, including Black Pepper in a formulation with Turmeric increases the bioavailability of curcumin, maximizing its anti-inflammatory effects.

Customizing Combinations for Individual Needs

- **Personal Health Profiles**: Consider the unique health needs and conditions of the individual when creating herbal combinations. Customize formulations to address specific health issues, allergies, or sensitivities.

- **Adjusting Dosages**: Tailor the dosages of each herb in a combination based on their potency and the individual's health requirements. This ensures optimal effectiveness and safety of the formulation.

- **Feedback and Iteration**: Collect feedback on the effectiveness of your herbal combinations and be prepared to adjust formulations based on results. This iterative process helps refine your products to better meet the needs of users.

Conclusion

Combining herbs for enhanced effects is a powerful strategy in herbal medicine, allowing you to create formulations that are greater than the sum of their parts. By understanding herbal synergy, balancing actions, and customizing combinations for specific health needs, you can develop effective herbal tablets that provide comprehensive and targeted benefits. This approach not only enhances the potency of your products but also ensures they are safe, effective, and tailored to meet the diverse needs of your users.

Troubleshooting Common Issues

Creating herbal tablets at home can sometimes come with challenges, especially if you are new to herbal medicine or tablet formulation. This section provides practical solutions to common problems you may encounter while making herbal tablets, ensuring that your formulations are effective, safe, and of high quality.

Tablet Binding Problems

- **Issue: Tablets are Crumbling or Falling Apart**

  - **Cause**: This often occurs when there is not enough binding agent in the mixture or when the herbs used are too coarse. The binding agent helps the powdered herbs adhere to each other and form a solid tablet.

  - **Solution**: Increase the amount of binding agent, such as acacia gum, maltodextrin, or a natural syrup. Also, ensure that the herbs are finely ground to a powder. A finer consistency allows for better cohesion when pressed into tablets.

- **Issue: Tablets are Too Hard or Difficult to Swallow**

  - **Cause**: Too much binding agent or compressing the tablets too tightly can result in excessively hard tablets.

  - **Solution**: Reduce the amount of binding agent or adjust the pressure used in the tablet press. Experiment with different levels of compression until you find a balance that produces a solid but not overly hard tablet.

Problems with Herb Quality and Potency

- **Issue: Tablets are Not Effective**

  - **Cause**: The herbs used may not be fresh, potent, or properly stored. Additionally, incorrect dosages or combinations could reduce effectiveness.

  - **Solution**: Ensure you are using high-quality, fresh herbs sourced from reputable suppliers. Store herbs properly in airtight containers away from light, heat, and moisture. Review the formulation to ensure the correct dosages and effective combinations of herbs are being used.

- **Issue: Unpleasant Taste or Smell**

- **Cause**: Some herbs naturally have strong, unpleasant tastes or odors that can be off-putting.

- **Solution**: Use flavor-masking agents like mint or licorice root powder, or coat tablets with a thin layer of honey or plant-based sweetener. You can also try encapsulating the tablets in a vegetable-based capsule to mask the taste and smell.

Issues with Tablet Appearance and Consistency

- **Issue: Tablets are Sticking to the Press or Molding Equipment**

  - **Cause**: This can happen if the mixture is too moist or if the tablet press is not properly lubricated.

  - **Solution**: Ensure the herbal mixture has the correct moisture content—not too wet or too dry. Use a natural lubricant, such as vegetable oil, on the tablet press to prevent sticking.

- **Issue: Uneven Tablet Sizes or Shapes**

  - **Cause**: Uneven pressure during the pressing process or inconsistent measuring of ingredients can result in tablets of varying sizes and shapes.

- **Solution**: Use a precise measuring spoon or scale to ensure uniformity in the amount of herbal mixture used per tablet. Adjust the tablet press to apply even pressure across all tablets.

Storage and Shelf Life Challenges

- **Issue: Tablets Are Losing Potency Over Time**

  - **Cause**: Exposure to air, moisture, light, or heat can degrade the active compounds in herbal tablets.

  - **Solution**: Store tablets in airtight, opaque containers in a cool, dry place. Consider adding natural desiccants like silica gel packets to absorb any moisture and extend shelf life.

- **Issue: Tablets Are Developing Mold or Spoilage**

  - **Cause**: This can occur if the tablets are stored in a humid environment or if the herbs used were not properly dried.

  - **Solution**: Ensure that all herbs are thoroughly dried before use, and store the finished tablets in a cool, dry place. Consider vacuum sealing or using moisture-absorbing packets to further protect against humidity.

Formulation and Dosage Adjustments

- **Issue: Overdose or Side Effects from Tablets**

  - ○ **Cause**: Incorrect dosage calculations or improper combinations of herbs can lead to side effects or overdoses.

  - ○ **Solution**: Carefully research the recommended dosages for each herb and follow guidelines for safe combinations. Start with lower dosages and gradually increase as needed, observing for any adverse reactions.

- **Issue: Tablets Are Too Large or Difficult to Dose**

  - ○ **Cause**: Using too many ingredients or high dosages can result in large, hard-to-swallow tablets.

  - ○ **Solution**: Break down the formulation into smaller doses, spread across multiple tablets if needed. Alternatively, consider using smaller quantities of high-potency extracts to reduce the overall tablet size.

General Tips for Troubleshooting

- **Maintain a Detailed Log**: Keep track of all ingredients, dosages, and processes used in each batch of tablets. This log will help identify and correct issues in future batches.

- **Experiment and Adjust**: Herbal tablet-making is both a science and an art. Be prepared to experiment with different formulations, binders, and pressing techniques to achieve the desired results.

- **Seek Feedback**: If you are making herbal tablets for others, seek feedback on their effectiveness and any issues experienced. This will provide valuable insights for improving your formulations.

By understanding these common issues and their solutions, you can troubleshoot effectively and refine your herbal tablet-making process, ensuring high-quality, effective, and safe natural remedies.

Chapter 7: Integrating Herbal Tablets into Daily Life

Creating a Personal Herbal Tablet Routine

Establishing a personal herbal tablet routine is key to incorporating natural remedies into your daily life effectively. A consistent regimen ensures that you receive the full benefits of the herbs and helps you maintain optimal health. Here's how to create a personalized herbal tablet routine that aligns with your lifestyle and health goals:

Assess Your Health Needs

The first step in creating a routine is to assess your specific health needs. Consider the following questions:

- What are your primary health concerns? (e.g., digestive issues, stress, immune support)

- Are there any conditions you want to manage or prevent? (e.g., joint pain, cognitive decline)

- Do you have any allergies or sensitivities to certain herbs?

Identifying your health goals will help you select the right herbal tablets and create a regimen tailored to your needs.

Choose the Right Herbal Tablets

Based on your health assessment, choose the herbal tablets that best suit your needs. For example:

- **Immune Support**: Consider echinacea and elderberry tablets for enhancing your immune system.

- **Stress Relief**: Opt for ashwagandha or valerian root tablets to help manage stress and anxiety.

- **Digestive Health**: Use peppermint and ginger tablets to soothe digestive issues.

Ensure that the herbs you select are safe for you, especially if you are taking other medications or have underlying health conditions.

Determine the Optimal Dosage and Timing

Once you have chosen your herbal tablets, determine the optimal dosage and timing for each:

- **Morning Routine**: Take energizing herbs like ginseng or adaptogens like rhodiola in the morning to help boost energy and focus throughout the day.

- **Midday Support**: Digestive aids such as fennel or peppermint can be taken with lunch to support digestion and reduce bloating.

- **Evening Wind-Down**: Calming herbs like chamomile or passionflower are ideal for the evening to promote relaxation and improve sleep quality.

Following a structured timing plan will help you integrate herbal tablets into your routine without disrupting your daily activities.

Incorporate Herbal Tablets into Your Meals

To enhance absorption and make it easier to remember your doses, consider taking your herbal tablets with meals:

- **With Breakfast**: Start your day with energizing and immune-boosting herbs taken with a healthy breakfast.

- **With Lunch and Dinner**: Take digestive and anti-inflammatory tablets with your main meals to maximize their benefits.

- **Before Bed**: Consume calming or sleep-promoting tablets in the evening to prepare your body for restful sleep.

Incorporating tablets into your mealtime routine makes it easier to remember to take them consistently.

Adjust and Monitor Your Routine

Your herbal tablet routine should be flexible and adaptable to your changing health needs:

- **Start Slowly**: Begin with a lower dose to see how your body responds to each herb. Gradually increase the dosage as needed, based on the desired effects and any side effects you may experience.

- **Monitor Effects**: Keep a journal to track your progress, noting any changes in your symptoms, energy levels, mood, or overall well-being.

- **Make Adjustments**: Based on your observations, adjust the dosages or switch out herbs to better suit your needs. Consult with an herbalist or healthcare provider for guidance on making these adjustments safely.

Regularly monitoring your routine ensures that you are receiving the maximum benefits from your herbal tablets.

Sustain Your Routine with Practical Tips

Maintaining a consistent herbal tablet routine can be made easier with these practical tips:

- **Set Reminders**: Use a smartphone app or set alarms to remind you when to take your tablets.

- **Prepare in Advance**: Organize your tablets in a weekly pill organizer to streamline your daily routine.

- **Stay Informed**: Keep learning about the herbs you use and stay updated on any new findings or recommendations.

By integrating these strategies into your daily life, you can sustain a healthy herbal tablet routine that supports your wellness journey.

Creating a personal herbal tablet routine allows you to harness the power of natural remedies effectively, providing a structured approach to achieving your health goals. Tailoring your routine to your specific needs ensures that you receive the most benefit from the herbs, enhancing your overall quality of life.

Combining Tablets with Other Natural Remedies

To enhance the effectiveness of herbal tablets, consider combining them with other natural remedies. This holistic approach can provide comprehensive support for your health, targeting multiple aspects of wellness simultaneously. By integrating various natural therapies, you can create a well-rounded regimen that amplifies the benefits of each component. Here's how to effectively combine herbal tablets with other natural remedies:

Pairing Herbal Tablets with Teas

Herbal teas are a gentle and effective way to complement the benefits of herbal tablets. They provide hydration and deliver the therapeutic properties of herbs in a soothing form. For example:

- **Immune Support**: Pair echinacea tablets with a warm cup of elderberry or ginger tea to enhance immune function and provide additional antiviral support.

- **Digestive Health**: Combine peppermint or ginger tablets with fennel or chamomile tea to soothe digestive discomfort and reduce bloating.

- **Relaxation and Sleep**: Complement valerian root or ashwagandha tablets with a calming blend of chamomile and lavender tea in the evening to promote relaxation and restful sleep.

By pairing herbal tablets with teas, you can target specific health concerns more effectively while enjoying the comforting ritual of tea preparation.

Using Essential Oils Alongside Herbal Tablets

Essential oils offer concentrated plant extracts that can be used aromatically, topically, or in some cases, internally to enhance the effects of herbal tablets:

- **Stress Relief**: Use calming essential oils like lavender, chamomile, or frankincense in a diffuser or apply them topically to pulse points while taking stress-relief tablets like rhodiola or lemon balm.

- **Pain Management**: Complement anti-inflammatory tablets such as turmeric and ginger with essential oils like peppermint or eucalyptus applied topically to affected areas for additional pain relief.

- **Respiratory Support**: Combine respiratory-support tablets like eucalyptus or thyme with essential oil inhalation to open airways and enhance breathing.

Combining essential oils with herbal tablets creates a multi-sensory healing experience, providing both immediate and long-term benefits.

Integrating Herbal Tablets with Dietary Changes

Diet plays a crucial role in supporting the body's healing processes, and certain foods can enhance the effectiveness of herbal tablets:

- **Anti-Inflammatory Diet**: Complement anti-inflammatory tablets (like turmeric and boswellia) with a diet rich in anti-inflammatory foods, such as leafy greens, berries, and fatty fish.

- **Gut Health**: Enhance the effects of digestive support tablets (like peppermint and ginger) by consuming probiotic-rich foods (such as yogurt, kefir, or sauerkraut) and prebiotic fibers (found in bananas, onions, and garlic).

- **Detoxification**: Combine detox-supporting herbal tablets (such as dandelion or milk thistle) with a diet high in fiber, fresh fruits, and vegetables to aid in the body's natural detox processes.

Aligning your herbal regimen with a complementary diet can significantly boost your body's ability to heal and maintain balance.

Complementing Tablets with Physical Therapies

Physical therapies such as massage, acupuncture, or yoga can be excellent additions to a regimen that includes herbal tablets:

- **Pain and Inflammation**: Use herbal pain relief tablets (like willow bark or devil's claw) alongside regular massage therapy or acupuncture sessions to reduce pain and inflammation more effectively.

- **Stress and Anxiety**: Combine calming herbal tablets (such as passionflower or kava kava) with mindfulness practices like meditation, yoga, or tai chi to enhance relaxation and stress management.

- **Circulatory Health**: Pair cardiovascular-support tablets (like hawthorn or ginkgo biloba) with aerobic exercises, such as walking or cycling, to improve circulation and heart health.

Physical therapies can enhance the absorption and effectiveness of herbal tablets while supporting overall physical and mental well-being.

Combining Tablets with Tinctures and Extracts

Tinctures and extracts are potent liquid forms of herbs that can be used alongside tablets to provide a stronger therapeutic effect:

- **Targeted Health Issues**: Use an herbal tincture for acute issues, such as echinacea tincture for a sudden immune challenge, while taking herbal tablets for ongoing support.

- **Enhanced Potency**: For conditions requiring more intensive support, like chronic pain or severe anxiety, consider using both tablets and tinctures of the same herb for a more potent effect.

- **Convenient and Fast-Acting**: Tinctures are absorbed more quickly than tablets, providing a rapid onset of effects, which can be useful in acute situations.

By combining tablets with tinctures, you can tailor your herbal regimen to meet both immediate and long-term health needs.

Utilizing Herbal Tablets with Topical Remedies

Topical herbal remedies, such as salves, creams, and compresses, can be used alongside herbal tablets to provide localized relief:

- **Skin Health**: Pair skin-supporting tablets (like neem and aloe vera) with a topical cream containing calendula or tea tree oil for enhanced healing of skin conditions.

- **Muscle and Joint Pain**: Combine pain-relief tablets (such as turmeric and ginger) with a topical salve containing arnica or cayenne to reduce inflammation and pain locally.

- **Wound Healing**: Use wound-healing herbal tablets (like comfrey or gotu kola) in conjunction with topical applications of herbal antiseptics like yarrow or goldenseal.

Topical remedies can provide immediate, localized relief while the herbal tablets work systemically.

Creating a Comprehensive Natural Healing Plan

To create a holistic natural healing plan, integrate herbal tablets with other natural remedies, such as:

- **Lifestyle Practices**: Include regular physical activity, adequate hydration, and sufficient rest to support overall health.

- **Nutritional Support**: Ensure a balanced diet rich in nutrients that support herbal efficacy.

- **Mind-Body Techniques**: Incorporate mindfulness, meditation, or relaxation techniques to complement the calming effects of certain herbs.

By combining herbal tablets with a range of natural remedies, you create a comprehensive and balanced approach to health and wellness, enhancing the body's natural healing processes and supporting long-term vitality.

Case Studies and Success Stories

Including real-life case studies and success stories can provide readers with practical insights and inspiration on how to effectively use herbal tablets for natural healing. These stories highlight the transformative power of herbal remedies and demonstrate their application in everyday life. In this section, you will find a variety of case studies showcasing different health issues, the herbal tablets used, and the outcomes experienced by individuals.

Overcoming Chronic Pain with Herbal Tablets

Meet Jane, a 52-year-old woman who struggled with chronic joint pain due to arthritis. Despite trying various conventional treatments, she continued to suffer from debilitating pain. After consulting with an herbalist, Jane started taking a combination of turmeric and boswellia tablets, known for their anti-inflammatory properties. Within a few weeks, she noticed a significant reduction in pain and stiffness. With continued use, Jane was able to resume her daily activities without discomfort and reduce her reliance on over-the-counter pain medications.

Boosting Immune Health During Cold and Flu Season

Tom, a father of three, was constantly falling ill during the winter months, struggling with frequent colds and respiratory infections. Looking for a natural way to strengthen his immune system, he began taking a daily regimen of echinacea and elderberry tablets. After just one season, Tom noticed a marked improvement in his health; he had fewer colds and recovered more quickly when he did catch one. Encouraged by these results, he continued using herbal tablets as a preventive measure for his entire family.

Managing Anxiety Naturally

Emily, a 30-year-old professional, dealt with high levels of stress and anxiety due to her demanding job. Seeking a natural alternative to prescription medications, she explored the use of herbal tablets. Emily incorporated ashwagandha and valerian root tablets into her daily routine, along with mindfulness practices. Over the course of several months, Emily experienced a significant decrease in her anxiety levels and was able to manage her stress more effectively. The combination of herbal tablets and lifestyle changes provided her with a sustainable, holistic approach to mental well-being.

Supporting Digestive Health Through Natural Remedies

David, a 45-year-old businessman, frequently suffered from bloating and indigestion after meals. Frustrated with the lack of relief from conventional treatments, he turned to herbal medicine. David started using peppermint and ginger tablets, known for their digestive soothing effects. Within days, he noticed a reduction in his symptoms and an overall improvement in his digestive health. By maintaining this regimen, David was able to enjoy his meals without discomfort and felt more energetic throughout the day.

Hormonal Balance and Women's Health

Maria, a 38-year-old mother, faced hormonal imbalances after the birth of her second child, which caused irregular menstrual cycles and mood swings. After extensive research, she decided to try vitex and dong quai tablets, which are traditionally used to support hormonal balance. Within three months, Maria's cycles became more regular, and her mood swings were significantly reduced. She felt more in control of her health and empowered by the natural approach to managing her symptoms.

Enhancing Cognitive Function in Older Adults

John, a 67-year-old retiree, was concerned about age-related cognitive decline. Seeking a natural way to maintain his mental acuity, he began taking a combination of ginkgo biloba and lion's mane mushroom tablets, which are known for their brain-boosting properties. Over time, John noticed improvements in his memory and focus. His daily crossword puzzles became easier, and he felt more confident in his cognitive abilities, attributing these changes to the consistent use of herbal tablets.

Combating Skin Issues Naturally

Sarah, a 25-year-old with persistent acne and skin irritation, decided to try a natural approach after conventional treatments failed to produce long-lasting results. She started using a combination of neem and aloe vera tablets, which are known for their anti-inflammatory and skin-healing properties. Within weeks, Sarah noticed a visible reduction in acne and an overall improvement in her skin texture. She felt more comfortable in her skin and gained confidence as her complexion continued to clear.

Addressing Cardiovascular Health Concerns

Mark, a 55-year-old man with a family history of heart disease, wanted to take preventive measures to support his cardiovascular health. After consulting with a healthcare professional, he incorporated hawthorn berry and garlic tablets into his daily regimen. These herbs are recognized for their heart-supportive qualities, such as improving circulation and reducing cholesterol levels. After several months of use, Mark's blood pressure stabilized, and his cholesterol levels improved, demonstrating the efficacy of his natural approach.

Conclusion

These case studies and success stories serve as a testament to the power of herbal tablets in promoting natural healing and overall well-being. By sharing these real-life experiences, this book aims to inspire and guide readers in their journey towards better health through the use of herbal remedies. Whether dealing with chronic conditions or seeking preventive care, these stories highlight the versatility and effectiveness of herbal tablets as a natural alternative to conventional treatments.

Conclusion

In a world increasingly reliant on synthetic medications and treatments, the timeless wisdom of natural healing stands as a powerful alternative. **The Herbal Natural Plant Power Tablets Book: Your Complete Guide to Natural Healing** offers an extensive exploration into the world of herbal tablets, providing readers with the knowledge and tools necessary to harness the healing power of plants in a convenient, effective form.

Herbal tablets present a unique way to integrate the benefits of herbal medicine into daily life. They combine traditional knowledge with modern convenience, making them accessible for anyone seeking a more natural approach to health and wellness. From supporting the immune system to managing stress, pain, digestive issues, and more, herbal tablets offer a broad range of benefits with fewer side effects than many conventional medications.

Throughout this book, we've journeyed through the history, preparation, and application of herbal tablets, learning how to craft effective remedies for a wide variety of common health issues. We've delved into specialized formulations tailored to specific needs, explored advanced techniques for maximizing the potency of herbal preparations, and shared inspirational case studies showcasing the transformative impact of herbal tablets on people's lives.

This guide aims to empower you to take charge of your health naturally, offering clear instructions and practical advice on selecting, preparing, and using herbal tablets. Whether you are a seasoned herbalist or a beginner exploring natural remedies for the first time, this book provides a comprehensive foundation to help you make informed choices about your health and wellness.

As you continue your journey with herbal medicine, remember that each person's body is unique, and responses to herbs can vary. It is always advisable to consult with a healthcare professional, especially if you have underlying health conditions or are taking other medications. By combining knowledge, personal experience, and professional guidance, you can create a personalized approach to health that aligns with your needs and lifestyle.

Embrace the natural power of plants, and discover the benefits of herbal tablets as part of your daily health routine. May this book serve as a trusted companion on your path to natural healing and wellness. Remember, the power to heal and thrive lies within nature—and within you.

Made in the USA
Middletown, DE
30 August 2024

6004149OR00141